The Gene, the Clinic and the Family

T0075825

While some theorists argue that medicine is caught in a relentless process of 'geneticization' and others offer a thesis of biomedicalization, there is still little research that explores how these effects are accomplished in practice. Joanna Latimer, whose groundbreaking ethnography on acute health care organization and practice gave us the social science classic *The Conduct of Care*, moves her focus from the bedside to the clinic in this in-depth study of genetic medicine.

Against current thinking that proselytises the rise of laboratory science, Professor Latimer shows how the genetic clinic is at the heart of the revolution in the new genetics. Tracing how work on the abnormal in an embryonic genetic science, dysmorphology, is changing our thinking about the normal, *The Gene, the Clinic and the Family* charts new understandings about family, procreation and choice. Far from medicine experiencing the much-proclaimed 'death of the clinic', this book shows how medicine is both reasserting its status as a science and revitalising its dominance over society, not only for now but for societies in the future.

This book will appeal to students, scholars and professionals interested in medical sociology, science and technology studies, the anthropology of science, medical science and genetics, as well as genetic counselling.

Joanna Latimer is Professor of Sociology at Cardiff University School of Social Sciences, and Professor in the ESRC Centre for the Economic and Social Aspects of Genomics. She has been researching medical knowledge and practice ethnographically for 30 years. Professor Latimer is editor of *Sociology of Health and Illness*, a member of the board of *The Sociological Review*, and chair of the Cardiff Ageing, Science and Older People Network.

Genetics and Society

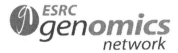

Series Editors:

Ruth Chadwick, *Director of Cesagen, Cardiff University*, John Dupré, *Director of Egenis, Exeter University*, David Wield, *Director of Innogen, Edinburgh University*, and Steve Yearley, *Director of the Genomics Forum, Edinburgh University*.

The books in this series, all based on original research, explore the social, economic and ethical consequences of the new genetic sciences. The series is based at Cesagen, one of the centres forming the ESRC's Genomics Network (EGN), the largest UK investment in social-science research on the implications of these innovations. With a mix of research monographs, edited collections, textbooks and a major new handbook, the series is a valuable contribution to the social analysis of developing and emergent bio-technologies.

Series titles include:

New Genetics, New Social Formations
Peter Glasner, Paul Atkinson and Helen Greenslade

New Genetics, New Identities
Paul Atkinson, Peter Glasner and Helen Greenslade

The GM Debate
Risk, politics and public engagement
Tom Horlick-Jones, John Walls, Gene Rowe, Nick Pidgeon, Wouter Poortinga, Graham Murdock and Tim O'Riordan

Growth Cultures
Life sciences and economic development
Philip Cooke

Human Cloning in the Media
Joan Haran, Jenny Kitzinger, Maureen McNeil and Kate O'Riordan

Local Cells, Global Science
Embryonic stem cell research in India
Aditya Bharadwaj and Peter Glasner

Handbook of Genetics and Society
Paul Atkinson, Peter Glasner and Margaret Lock

The Human Genome
Chamundeeswari Kuppuswamy

Community Genetics and Genetic Alliances
Eugenics, carrier testing and networks of risk
Aviad E. Raz

The Gene, the Clinic and the Family

Diagnosing dysmorphology, reviving medical dominance

Joanna Latimer

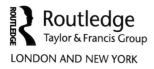

Routledge
Taylor & Francis Group

LONDON AND NEW YORK

First published 2013
by Routledge
2 Park Square, Milton Park, Abingdon, Oxfordshire OX14 4RN

Simultaneously published in the USA and Canada
by Routledge
711 Third Avenue, New York, NY 10017

First issued in paperback 2014

Routledge is an imprint of the Taylor & Francis Group, an informa business

© 2013 Joanna Latimer

The right of Joanna Latimer to be identified as author of this work has been
asserted by her in accordance with sections 77 and 78 of the Copyright,
Designs and Patents Act 1988.

All rights reserved. No part of this book may be reprinted or reproduced or
utilized in any form or by any electronic, mechanical, or other means, now
known or hereafter invented, including photocopying and recording, or in any
information storage or retrieval system, without permission in writing from the
publishers.

Trademark notice: Product or corporate names may be trademarks or registered
trademarks, and are used only for identification and explanation without intent to
infringe.

British Library Cataloguing in Publication Data
A catalogue record for this book is available from the British Library

Library of Congress Cataloging in Publication Data
Latimer, Joanna
The gene, the clinic and the family: diagnosing dysmorphology,
reviving medical dominance / Joanna Latimer
    pages cm. — (Genetics and society)
Includes bibliographical references and index
1. Medical genetics. 2. Abnormalities, Human—Genetics aspects. I. Title
RB155.L375 2013
616'.042—dc23   2012050058

ISBN 978-0-415-69928-0 (hbk)

ISBN 978-1-138-85881-7 (pbk)

ISBN 978-0-203-44145-9 (ebk)

Typeset in Times New Roman
by Deer Park Productions

For Rolland and our children Jamie and Arabella, whose own generation will be much affected by the trends addressed in this book.

Contents

Figures

Preface

This book is rather like the clinic: a space of crossing and translation, between medical sociology and science studies, both anthropological and sociological. Thus the book draws attention to and helps deconstruct the dichotomy between the laboratory and the clinic, and between science and medicine.

The book draws on 25 years as a medical sociologist, researching acute medicine, primary care, accident and emergency, intensive care, paediatric genetics, geriatric medicine and biomedical science. My 'ethnographic' immersion in medicine and health care practice, however, began earlier by working for ten years in the British National Health Service, as a cleaner and nursing auxiliary in a geriatric hospital before I trained and practiced as a nurse and ward sister in both acute and primary care settings. While my close reading of the discourses of science and medicine owes much to my original training in English at the University of London, I have tried never to lose my grounding in everyday practice, my experiences with patients and that eye for detail that served me so well in those early days.

The core research material comes from a longitudinal study of an evolving discursive practice in medical genetics known as dysmorphology. This is the study of abnormal forms, historically called congenital abnormalities. Thus the analysis of the book locates itself in those effects in persons identified as 'existing from birth' and as relating to genitus, or 'begetting'. As it happens, dysmorphology's roots are in paediatrics and the objects and subjects of clinical practice are mainly children and their families. Indeed many clinical geneticists I met were trained in paediatrics and the underpinning discourses in the clinic are the science of growth and form in humans, such as embryology, and conceptions of child development.

Critically, dysmorphology is concerned with the description and recognition of 'syndromes'. At the time of the study there were over 3,000 syndromes recorded in databases, and many of these descriptions were still in the making. So the book is to some extent about shape and form in contemporary medicine, and, further, how deviations from normal human development are being identified and named. 'Dysmorph' literally means misshapen, and is concerned with begetting when the processes of reproduction go wrong and do so in ways that produce abnormal forms. It should be noted that these syndromes typically involve very small numbers of people, and come under the new rubric rare disorders. Consequently, the availability of molecular and cytogenic tests was limited.

The field of dysmorphology is also emerging at a time, the second decade of the new millennium, when biological understandings of the genetic and the congenital are changing and shifting. Hence dysmorphology is also busy relocating in relation to those understandings. Like biology, and no doubt because of its direct links to the biology of human development (specifically growth and form), dysmorphology is becoming more and more engrossed in the correlations between the genetic and deviations in growth and form. In so doing, dysmorphologists claim to be helping to shape the science of human development. So the first story I have to tell is about how the relations between medicine and science, the clinic and the gene, are in the process of being constructed in dysmorphology and in genetic medicine.

We might think these syndromes may simply represent difference – difference in one set of children and their parents from another; that where these differences are associated with pathology and reconstituted as problematic, what we have is a case study of abnormality or deviation that walks the tightrope of identity politics. What emerges however is how the genetics of normal human development relies on this mapping of deviations in growth and form, with the observation and description of congenital abnormality. So much so, that what seems to be evident is that it is the normal that is itself shrinking. As one geneticist put it to me: from his perspective, we all have a syndrome.

What is extraordinary to me is how in these new kinds of medical entities, syndromes, something so tiny as genetic mutation is being held responsible for the extraordinary disruption seen in some children's physical and intellectual growth and development, and across so many of their bodies' systems. This brings me to the second story I have to tell, which is about how we are all becoming drawn into these studies on growth and form and, further, how the findings in dysmorphology are likely to affect choice of partners and alter decisions about procreation in the future. The critical issue is thus of grasping the significance of these imaginaries – syndromes and other forms of classification – through which forms of life get constituted as malformations; and, understand when and why they bother us, literally and conceptually. What matters is what we do with these imaginaries, particularly in terms of ideas of family and relatedness, of personhood and conceptions of what it is to be human.

A third story concerns my interest in how medical power works. What I help to show, contrary to the predictions of other observers, is how medicine is retaining its dominance in society partly through the clinic. In a large part this has involved me in recognizing that the power of medicine rests not so much in its ability to help generate cures – important as these discoveries are – but rather in its sticking to classification and the method of doubt as forming the twin bases of science. What I hope to show is that medical power works as much through deferral as decision, and that this is what helps to retain the clinic – with its intimate links to the family – as the final arbiter.

All three stories I have to tell draw from formal fieldwork, but are tempered by what Anthony Cohen (1992) calls 'post-fieldwork fieldwork'. The earlier fieldwork included observation of clinical process and practice across a regional genetics service, observation of local, national and international academic meetings such as the London Dysmorphology Club, at which dysmorphologists present their cases, there are formal and informal interviews with leading experts in dysmorphology, examinations of dysmorphologists' papers and websites, syndrome websites and interviews with family members in their homes. Much of this was undertaken in collaboration with other researchers and I have also been working closely with biologists and geneticists on another study that has influenced my interpretation and understanding of the present material.

Throughout the book I have illustrated the text with the kinds of images used by dysmorphologists to help get readers inside the world dysmorphologists both inhabit and help create. This is because dysmorphology is 'very visual' in its procedures – and because each syndrome has its own special 'face'. Many of these images include the actual faces of babies and children; these actual faces being what clinicians call 'representative subjects'. While I have not specifically analysed each image, my analysis of the social, cultural and existential significance of the visual practices of this world appears in Chapters 9 and 10.

A book like this is, of course, not possible without enormous help from others. My thanks, and huge gratitude, are first due to all the families, doctor-scientists and nurses whose lives and work informed this book. I must also warmly thank my collaborators in the initial study, Paul Atkinson, Angus Clarke and Daniella Pilz, as well as Katie Featherstone, the research fellow on the study – although I should stress that they are not responsible for the analysis I present here, nor do they necessarily agree with my findings.

The following people at many different times and in many different ways have also given valuable commentary, support and encouragement: Barbara Adam, Huw Beynon, Ruth Chadwick, Adele Clarke, Emma Clavering, Sophie Davies, Yulia Egorova, Faye Ginsberg, Adam Hedgecoe, Alexandra Hillman, William Housley, Rachel Hurdley, Illana Löwy, Janice MacLaughlin, Mike Michael, Mara Miele, Dimitris Papadopoulos, Maria Puig de la Bellacasa, Paul Rabinow, Rayna Rapp, Michael Schillmeier, Bev Skeggs, Gareth Thomas and Paul White.

Marilyn Strathern as ever informs, reforms and shifts my perspective. I am also most grateful to the Economic and Social Research Council (ESRC) which funded the initial fieldwork and have supported me as a member of the Centre for Economic and Social Aspects of Genomics (Cesagen) for the last three years. I would also like to record how much I appreciate the ongoing scientific education I am being given by the zoologist, ecologist, geneticist, photographer, wit and friend, David Kipling, and note the importance of being introduced to the Philosophy and Epistemology of Science in the ESRC doctoral programme at the University of Edinburgh. Finally, where would I be without my husband, the philosopher Rolland Munro? Not anywhere very interesting, that is for sure. I also need to thank both him, and my daughter, Arabella, for their spectacular editorial work on the final draft of the book, as well as my son, Jamie, for helping me keep body and soul together throughout its conception.

Part I

Introduction and background

1 Introduction

> [T]he new genetics will prove to be an infinitely greater force for reshaping society and life than was the revolution in physics, *because it will be embedded throughout the social fabric at the microlevel by medical practices and a variety of other discourses.*
>
> (Rabinow 1992, p.241, emphasis added, by permission of Zone Books)

The new genetics promises great things: things that are absolutely central to the Euro-American pre-occupation with health, wealth and longevity. Indeed, only two decades since Paul Rabinow made this prediction about the new genetics 'reshaping society and life', its impact on society is already being felt everywhere: in food, in clothing, in politics, in lifestyle, and in health care. So much so that it seems safe to say the new genetics is already having this 'infinitely greater' impact on society than the revolution in physics accomplished. But how is this happening? And what exactly is the place of medicine in all this?

Analysts used to argue that medicine drew its authority and power from its jurisdiction over acute illness, enacting the heroic saving of lives rather than engaging with everyday ailments. This line of analysis was crucial in cementing understandings of what sociologists and anthropologists described as medical dominance. This is the view that, of all the professions, medicine had the greatest influence; and, further, that its consequent shaping of society was pervasive and profound. This was not merely to note that doctors were pre-eminent in rank, say to lawyers and accountants, or simply to recognise that health care systems, such as the British National Health Service, are the largest employers in the world. It is to hold that the very fabric and mores of our social institutions, including government as well as family, have been radically, if surreptitiously, altered by the ideas, methods and practices of medicine.

Yet this idea of medicine as a cultural and economic powerhouse was not to last. According to Olshansky and Carnes (2001), an earlier revolution in longevity involved technologies that radically changed how we live in terms of sanitation, diet and so forth. These gave us progressive control over 'environmental sources of mortality, but which had nothing to do with our basic biology' (p.84). These changes permitted a 'relatively unprecedented number of people to enter into the relatively unexplored older regions of the lifespan' with the consequence of this being a transition to 'causes of death that arise from flaws, breakdowns, and failures of the biological processes within our bodies' (p.84).

By the end of the 20th century the big story had changed in both politics as well the academy, recounting instead how medicine is now emasculated in the face of the long term, chronic disorders and degenerative illnesses of the West. Populations in Western nations might be living longer, but the aged are consequently plagued with expensive chronic and degenerative diseases that drain their wealth as well as their health. As Bech, the hero of John Updike's trilogy, states 'If the muggers don't get your wallet, the nursing homes will' (1998, p.32).

In this scenario of incurable cancers, and a multiplicity of diseases affecting those living longer, doctors are portrayed as reduced to little more than an administrative role of delivering protocols that have been devised elsewhere. In their place, a motley crew of other professions, including carers, dieticians, homeopaths, nurse practitioners, physiotherapists, and lifestyle gurus – even patients themselves – are becoming the indispensible experts for people to go to for therapy and solace.

A new frontier?

Against this prospect of a terminal decline in the influence of medicine, the new genetics augurs a new and very different frontier. The prospect before us is that interventions at the level of the genes offer solutions to problems Western medicine once saw as intractable:

> Nature is fallible and her works are imperfect. Human beings are no exception; our bodies decay and perish and our powers are limited. Seemingly from the beginning, human beings have been alive to the many ways in which what we have been given falls short of what we can envision and what we desire.
> (President's Council on Bioethics 2003a, p.1)

Contrastingly to this background, the new genetics is haunted by eugenic dreams of eliminating diseases as part of its mission to eradicate all physical and mental disability. Some of these interventions involve old technologies – such as prenatal testing for hereditary and other congenital disorders and termination of pregnancy – and even forms of therapy (Kass 2002). However, since the emergence of the new genetics, more radical interventions being contemplated seem almost god-like in their will to go well beyond selection techniques that supposedly procure better children:

> We are human, but can imagine gods. We die, but can imagine immortality. But human beings have more than longings and imaginations. Although we are far from omnipotent, we have extraordinary powers, unique among the earth's creatures, to shape our environment and even ourselves according to our wills.
> (President's Council on Bioethics 2003a, p.1)

Interventions in this re-making of the human involve the genetic engineering of embryos, or 'reprogenetics' (Pray 2008), technologies that alter a person's genetic makeup, as well as the development of personalised, tailor-made biomedicines that literally reorder behaviour (Hedgecoe 2004b). These possibilities range from interfering directly with disordered bodies – for instance by putting a stop on the reproduction of faulty genes – to more indirect changes – by, say, reproducing genetically compatible donors or even by inventing ways to modify and engineer the genes themselves.

Discoveries and technologies associated with the new genetics thus open up, among other things, possibilities for overcoming the intractable chronic and degenerative disorderings of Western bodies and minds. There is also much discussion for instance of the 'farming' of replacement body parts, as well as talk of finding ways to 'switch' the genes that power the ageing process and chronic diseases, turning them on and off like lights (e.g. Wynford-Thomas 2003).

In this tsunami of discovery there is continuous debate over the profound questions that arise as a consequence of the new genetics. Specifically, many questions address the issue as to whether or not we *should* condone this pursuit of enhancement:

> It is perhaps not surprising, therefore, that also from the beginning human beings have struggled with two opposing responses to our lot. Should we try to mould the imperfection we have been given into something closer to our ideal? Or should we content ourselves with beholding and enjoying it as it is? And what about our own natures? Does our ability to flourish as human beings depend on our ability to improve upon the human form or function? Or might the contrary be true: does our flourishing depend on accepting – or even celebrating – our natural limitations?
>
> (President's Council on Bioethics 2003b, p.1)

As this book will show, it is not enough to raise these questions in the abstract. Room has also to be given to explore, in depth, how the potential of the new genetics is also changing the very nature of what we view to be human. I then go on to discuss that, if claims about the new genetics are to carry, and the promises and hopes of enhancement bear fruit, there is also going to be a radical shift in the ways in which diseases and bodily 'disorderings' are represented and classified.

The alignment of clinical medicine with the new genetics

This is where the story of this book begins. Far from becoming relegated to being the handmaiden of genetic science – trained technicians applying the instructions on the pack – doctors and medical researchers are busy surfing these waves of innovation and making themselves pivotal to decisions as to who (or what) should be enhanced. Or, indeed, disposed of.

My adoption of Rabinow's prediction as the epigraph for this chapter is thus not simply to highlight the advent of the new genetics, whose importance today is hardly in dispute even when its more fanciful claims are dismissed. Rather the point is to draw the reader's attention to the explanation Rabinow offers for the impact of the new genetics on society overshadowing the revolution in physics. What Rabinow anticipates is that, in order to have any real impact, the new genetics needs to 'be embedded throughout the social fabric at the microlevel'. Critically, as Rabinow points out, this embedding will be accomplished by '*medical practices and a variety of other discourses*' (emphasis in the original).

A highly respected cultural anthropologist before he turned his attention to science and medicine, Rabinow is emphasizing medicine as the agent by which the much heralded changes in the new genetics become embedded in the social fabric. For it is medical practice, rather than ideas of genetics themselves, that he argues will transform society. What he clues us into is the obvious fact that the new genetics cannot work alone. It must align itself with medicine if it is to rework society in the various ways the pundits anticipate.

The statement by Rabinow cited at the opening of this chapter therefore invites reconsideration of a profound and long-standing relation: that which is established between medicine and society. This is after all his key point: medicine does not simply serve society. Medicine, particularly in the form Rabinow calls biomedicine, reforms and changes the social. Simply put, medicine *dominates* society.

In all this Rabinow has been more prescient than others in his anticipation of what the new genetics will accomplish. Against stories of a decline in the importance of medicine, including its geneticization and molecularization augured by, amongst others, Nikolas Rose (2007b), Rabinow's signal contribution is to identify the means by which the new genetics will reshape society and life – and so alert us to the conditions of possibility for this reshaping.

My own contribution is to go further than Rabinow. I demonstrate that the means by which the new genetics is reshaping society and life involve an extension and revitalization of the work of medicine. Indeed, as I go on to show, there is also what I am calling a 'rebirth' of the clinic.

Medicine and its engrossment

The present book addresses this question of the relation between medicine and the 'new genetics'. I am doing so at the end of the first decade of a new millennium, a time when genetics has been rapidly changing itself in light of the emergence of post-genomic biology. Significantly, where recent commentators have focussed on the relation between medicine and science, they have tended to beg the question in failing to examine medicine's own scientific standing.

This debate about medicine's relation to science is particularly lively in the context of assertions about the relationship between the laboratory – as the site of science on the one hand – and the clinic – as the site of medicine on the other – in what has been termed the 'geneticization' of medicine (Abbey Lipman in Miller 1999). Such assertions invite a potentially false dichotomy between the laboratory and the clinic in order to separate science from medicine. Some pundits also rely on the dubious notion that we are witnessing the passing of modernity, a contemporary decline of the power of rationalism and science (Ballard and Elston 2005, drawing on Schneider 2003) that leads to our putting our faith in alternatives to medical power.

To the contrary, I show how the reviving of medical power is made possible through contemporary conditions that speak for the intensification, not the waning, of all that is modern. As I explain later in detail, what makes medicine a science is the same as what keeps it modern: it is the construction of systematic forms of classification that can be used to 'categorize' persons. It is the work of classification that requires science to be conducted within the walls of the clinic – and in the presence of the persons being so classified – that makes glib separations of medicine from science so palpably false.

In this book I will unfold a somewhat different view to those held by theorists such as Rabinow, arguing that medicine engrosses itself through keeping the clinic as key to science and, through this engrossment, makes itself indispensible to both science and society. Much as money expands an economy and, in so doing, 'grows' our dependence upon it, medicine advises us over how we are to see the world and directs us over what is to be valued.

Since the 19th century, if not before, medicine has made the clinic the 'obligatory passage' (Latour 1987) in exercising its expertise over the identification of health need. As the fieldwork I draw on demonstrates, this is because it is medicine – not the biological sciences – which defines when, and at what moments, something constitutes a need in people. This is proving to be as true today as it has been for almost the last two centuries. The research I draw on illustrates how doctors may do this work of categorization in different ways, but underlines how they continue to accomplish their classifications on persons *in the realm of the clinic*.

Consequently, as I go on to show, it is through the clinic that the new genetics must pass in order to have any real impact on society. This categorical work of the clinic is thus infrastructural to the organization of not just health care systems, such as the NHS, but also to body–world relations, and ideas of personhood, identity and belonging (Latimer 1999, 2004, 2011). That is, in providing 'categories' for people to understand the vectors and limits under which their lives are being lived, medicine is doing much more in the clinic than merely riding the wave train generated by the seismic progress of the new genetics. Indeed, through its processes of classification, far from medicine being made redundant, its key institution – the clinic – is at the heart of the seismic activity of the genetic.

Identifying the pathological

In entering this realm of the clinic, I shadowed doctors and observed how they distinguish and differentiate what they see. In so doing I followed them as they uncovered the manifold varieties of the pathological.

The term pathological here is being used in the everyday, implicit and taken-for-granted sense of medical practice, not in reference to the domain of laboratory-based sciences of pathology (Atkinson 1995; Mol 2000, 2002). That is, I am using it to denote those processes at the heart of the medical matter when the effects someone displays are figured as signs of something *clinically wrong* with a person (which may or may not be corroborated by laboratory and other investigations). By way of example, you may go to your doctor with a rash that is red and itchy. To the doctor, this symptom is not yet a sign of a disease. For the rash to be translated into a sign, for it to have the impetus to be treated as the sign of a disease, the doctor must be able to 'see' it, potentially at least, as pathological. This seeing is a process of *establishing* the significance of the rash.

Identifying something as potentially 'pathological' is a corollary of what clinicians call 'differential diagnosis'. This is the process through which they name and identify the signs and symptoms someone displays as belonging to one or another diagnostic category; *or not*. There may be tests that can be done as a part of establishing whether or not a symptom is indeed a sign. These may include an intensification of the inspecting gaze through technologies of visualization – such as x-rays and scans, as well as measurements, such as blood and other pathological tests. But each of these also requires interpretation. It is through these diagnostic processes that people are included and excluded from a diagnostic category.

As I show throughout the book, in this work of differentiating the pathological, medicine is conducting a form of *identity work* on persons that leads on to admitting people to, or excluding them from, diagnostic categories. Think back to the red and itchy rash: given the apprehension that it may be the sign of something more, there is a mixture of relief and displacement when the doctor says, after questioning, that it is probably to do with your washing powder or shower gel. You are so ready to offer up accounts – protestations that you have never had any allergies or trouble before, how you have been to the pharmacy and used their recommended anti-itching creams, how you have altered your diet and tried changing your washing power, washing-up liquid, shampoo, shower gel and so on. You have your arm on display: the red itchy rash is plain to see. You are full of apprehension, anticipation and hope. These only to be dashed as the doctor sends you home with no diagnosis: the move disposes you and the rash – there is nothing pathological there, it isn't, yet at least, a *clinical problem*. The clinic is thus both a moment of immersion in the real – 'look here it is, my arm, red, and itchy' – and a site of agonistics (Latimer 2004; Lyotard 1984) of who or what can account for the underpinnings of the real.

Please do not mistake me here as saying the categorical work of the clinic is purely clinical; as other studies have shown, diagnostic work serves and is effected by many agendas (Berg 1992; Dingwall and Murray 1983; Hillman *et al.* 2010; Latimer 1997). Rather, my point is that these processes of inclusion and exclusion in what counts as pathological are central to medicine's claim to being a science. The diagnostic categories constitute the 'categorical work' of medicine: it is the *realm* of what is sometimes referred to as 'clinical judgement' and is *the* domain of the clinic. And, critically, this centrality of classification is as much about doubt, and the precarious nature of diagnosis, as it is about certainty.

There is always a tension between the existence of doubt and the desire for certainty (Charon and Wyer 2008), a tension that, I suggest, opens up and institutes an endless demand for medical discretion and judgement.

The everyday work of establishing whether or not something is pathological, and of inclusion and exclusion to and from diagnostic categories in the clinic, is therefore key to understanding medical power as a particular form of power, which revolves around the retention and redistribution of *discretion*. As I go on to show not only do clinicians transform themselves into 'centres of discretion' (Munro 1999a) by transferring much of the discretion in diagnosis from the patient to themselves, they also retain discretion in diagnosis by postponing the meaning of laboratory findings back to their clinical judgement.

Power and deferral

It is helpful before continuing to emphasize that the site under study has two interdependent interfaces. The first interface takes place between the institutions of genetic technoscience and clinical medicine, namely the laboratory and the clinic, and between the participants therein, namely the biologist and the doctor. The second interface is between the clinic and that other key social institution, the family. It is here that the classification practices of medicine are not only put into practice, but are themselves being constructed and reconstructed by way of interchanges and interactions between the doctor and the patients.

Understanding the clinic as a 'centre of discretion' refers to the first of these two interfaces and helps balance off Bruno Latour's (1987) exegesis of the laboratory as a 'centre of calculation'. Power is never mastered though measurement alone. While it is certainly the case that much measurement has moved from the clinic to the laboratory, calculation for Latour means both measurement *and* decision.

For the clinicians to retain power it is necessary for there to be processes of deferral that return decision-making to the clinic. It is crucial to medicine's fate that its arrangements *defer* the moment of decision away from laboratory results. For all the measurements in the laboratory, this aspect of calculation must wait upon the discretion of clinicians. Crucial to medicine retaining its power is the mundane fact that this identity work of categorizing persons is never finalised ahead of the consultation with the family in the clinic.

We need to be careful with what we think is going on here. This is not just me observing an everyday form of deferral that proceeds by way of patients granting authority to clinicians – giving way as in the case of the rash discussed above to those who hold themselves out to have knowledge that we ourselves do not possess. This latter form of deferral, akin to agricultural labourers doffing their cap to the farmer, is certainly a mainstay of the second kind of interface – relations between the clinic and the family. But it is, in the dysmorphology clinic at least, not entirely a one-way street. As I hope to show, that something is or is not pathological (and that it then belongs or doesn't to a diagnostic category) has also to be made to hold in the clinic in the face of potentially contradictory evidence that comes from the family, not just the laboratory.

Bringing these two interfaces into consideration with one another helps to explain how medicine orders and re-orders scientific work in the laboratory. Only at the moment of diagnosis is 'opinion' delivered, consecrating the patient as having (or not having) this or that pathology; and as belonging (or not belonging) to this or that diagnostic category. Even after this consecration, there is room for doubt. After all, what has been delivered to patients in the context of the clinic remains, expressly, an opinion! Medicine always holds itself out as ready for a 'second opinion'. Doctors are not automatons and a different doctor may disagree, exercising what I am going to be calling their 'powers of discretion'. As I show throughout the book, this deferral of knowledge to the clinical moment is absolutely key to medicine's power. It is this process of deferral that keeps the clinic pivotal – not only to the integration of genetic science with society – but because it makes the family the essential point of delivery, and discovery, of scientific knowledge in human genetics.

The culture of enhancement

A key focus on these two interfaces is the emergent space of what Adele Clarke and her colleagues (2003, 2010) call biomedicalization, an era of even more intense medicalization covering all aspects of life, health and death. In unpicking this thesis of biomedicalization, and showing the extent to which medical dominance has never really declined, it is necessary to watch closely how ideas, as well as people's bodies and their parts, travel backwards and forwards between these two interfaces for examination, categorization and intervention.

To fulfil its promise, the new genetics has not only to understand the molecular basis of disease: it has to crash through the barriers constructed around the current reality of greater longevity being drained of health and wealth by chronic and degenerative illness. This is why the promise of the new genetics sits so well with, and indeed is so very much a part of a culture of enhancement, in which technoscience is figured as empowering and enabling (Strathern 1995, 1996).

Yet all this promise rests upon medical practitioners re-representing the *origins* of disease and disorders of the body, their aetiologies and natural histories, *as* genetic, rather than as the effects of lifestyle or environment. As illustrated in the example I give next of a syndrome, there have to be practices of distinction through which particular effects found in bodies can be ascribed as having a *genetic* origin. That is, there needs to be a subterranean shift in the grounds of explanation, and aetiology, of disease, and in the very ways in which phenomena are identified and categorized as clinically pathological. The proposed causes of ill health, disability and disease have to change.

In order to be persuasive, these new grounds of explanation must be compelling. As at the same time as authoritative statements circulate about what is already known, they must also be inventive – offering something new that gives hope. So shifts in explanatory grounds need to occur not only within medicine itself, but also in society, particularly in terms of how people imagine themselves and appear to each other.

As I go on to show, for all that dysmorphology begins with the abnormal, these shifts are likely to end up affecting a much wider array of persons. There are changes afoot in terms of how both doctors and ordinary people imagine the origins of how our bodies look or function. The various chapters in this book draw on my field study of dysmorphology to explore how this subterranean shift is being accomplished. What is changing are ideas about what it is that makes up the normal as well as the abnormal; and, of course, with this, the categories that make up the pathological.

Dysmorphology: a study in medical power

Am I being nostalgic in hanging onto the notion of the clinic and its intimate relations with the family? As already mentioned, views that champion the laboratory as the key site of the new genetics beg the question of how medicine might be in a better position to embed the new genetics into society, to say nothing of the vexed issue of medical dominance. Nonetheless, it is fair to question the place of the family here. Could social life really be reshaped by an alliance of the laboratory and the clinic that by-passes the family and makes medicine entirely beholden to the new genetics?

To ground my themes of medical power in an empirical field, and avoid the kind of abstraction that too often glosses over the intricacies and complexities involved, I draw on a field study of dysmorphology throughout the book. The fieldwork for this study tracked dysmorphology through all its interfaces, alignments, occasions, discourses, processes, practices and technologies.

The clinical definition of dysmorphology is the professional discipline of delineating disorders affecting the physical development of individuals, before or after birth (Aase 1990). In Europe dysmorphology has evolved as a sub-discipline, or knowledge practice, within medical or human genetics. Importantly for understanding how dysmorphology works as a science, classification takes place not in the diagnosis of diseases, but in terms of *syndromes*.

Here is a brief example of the kind of talk by experts which illustrates their focus on syndromes:

DR CASEY, SPECIALIST REGISTRAR IN GENETIC MEDICINE: He's [Simon] an autistic boy, very autistic. They [Simon's parents] need a long chat.

DR SMITH, CONSULTANT GENETICIST: Yes … I am just wondering if he should remind me of anything. (Pause). Not at the moment.

DR CASEY: A lot of it [medical perception in dysmorphology] is pattern recognition.

DR SMITH: The only other thing. He wasn't typical; he was too like his family. I'm always very cautious.

DR CASEY: We've all got a syndrome.

DR SMITH: Yes, we have a unique syndrome. There is a condition with fleshy earlobes but he didn't even have constipation problems so we can't go down that route. [They both look at their notes.]

DR CASEY: I know what I am thinking of – Coffin-Lowry; they tend to have cone-shaped epiphyses, but he's not hyperteloric [widely spaced eyes] enough.[1]

In what kind of classificatory system do 'fleshy earlobes' sit alongside 'constipation'? And how would 'widely spaced eyes' be significant? How can someone like Simon not be 'typical' (of what? a syndrome?) and yet be 'too like' his family? And what does it mean that a syndrome is something we all have, something that is unique to each of us? Can we 'be' a syndrome that is unique, but also belong to another kind of syndrome that is shared, like Coffin-Lowry?

It is striking that these doctors are not talking about a disease – diseases are something that people or their bodies have: someone has meningitis, or cancer, or multiple sclerosis. These doctors are talking differently. Critically, a syndrome is both something that someone is, and/or belongs to.

So what is a 'syndrome'? Syndromes are combinations and associations between diseases, and other signs and symptoms, including unusual features, which may or may not represent pathologies or deformities. They are 'associations', a 'concourse' of things, that live alongside each other, or fit together. For example, Coffin-Lowry syndrome is described as:

> a rare genetic disorder characterized by craniofacial (head and facial) and skeletal abnormalities, mental retardation, short stature, and hypotonia. Characteristic facial features may include an underdeveloped upper jaw bone (maxillary hypoplasia), a broad nose, protruding nostrils (nares), an abnormally prominent brow, downslanting eyelid folds (palpebral fissures), widely spaced eyes (hypertelorism), large ears, and unusually thick eyebrows. Skeletal abnormalities may include abnormal front-to-back and side-to-side curvature of the spine (kyphoscoliosis), unusual prominence of the breastbone (pectus carinatum), and short, hyperextensible, tapered fingers. Additional abnormalities may also be present. Other features may include feeding and respiratory problems, developmental delay, mental retardation, hearing impairment, awkward gait, flat feet, and heart and kidney involvement. The disorder affects males and females in equal numbers, however, symptoms may be more severe in males. Females may show mild mental retardation. The disorder is caused by a defective gene, RSK2, which was found in 1996 on the X chromosome (Xp22.2-p22.1). The gene codes for a member of a growth factor regulated protein kinase. It is unclear how changes (mutations) in the DNA structure of the gene lead to the clinical findings.
>
> (National Institute of Neurological Disorders and Stroke, undated)

Many syndromes like Coffin-Lowry have a particular look or 'face'. Figure 1.1 shows a 'picture' of Davis James Illa. His photograph is reproduced with kind permission of his mother, Mary C. Hoffman, Founder of the Coffin-Lowry Syndrome Foundation. The family portrait of James doubles as a clinical picture of someone whom clinicians call a 'representative subject': they have the typical face and features of the syndrome.

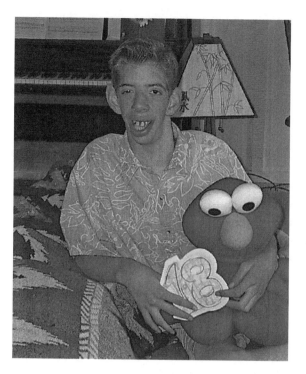

Figure 1.1 Welcome to the Coffin Lowry Syndrome Website. Reproduced with kind permission of Mary C. Hoffman, founder of the Coffin-Lowry Syndrome Foundation.

The picture is also on the Coffin-Lowry Syndrome Foundation webpage – described as a resource for families, teachers, relatives and clinicians:

> Welcome to The Coffin-Lowry Syndrome Foundation (CLSF). The purpose of CLSF is to provide a clearinghouse for information on Coffin-Lowry Syndrome (CLS), and to provide families affected by CLS a general forum in which to exchange information, ideas and advice. CLSF provides family matching services, telephone support, online discussion forum, an informational database and publishes an on-line newsletter, CLSF News. The newsletter is available in hard-copy free of charge to members without internet access. The online discussion forum is restricted to families, caregivers, teachers and medical professionals who have direct connections with CLS individuals.
>
> (Coffin-Lowry Syndrome Foundation, undated)

Classification in dysmorphology proceeds, not in terms of diseases, but *syndromes*, which includes both pathological and non-pathological signs and features. What I want to stress here is that people like James in the photograph cannot simply enter the clinic and hold out or point to the part of them that isn't working properly – the rash on their arm, for example. There is nothing pathological about James' face in itself, albeit that the photograph of him has become representative of the diagnostic category that he has in common with some others.

Pathology at the genetic level is productive of syndromes, and syndromes are holistic – they work across systems – and are something that someone is. But they may also be more than this. They may also be something that a family is. Thus diagnostic categories are very complex and – as can be seen from the above description of Coffin-Lowry syndrome – associated with genetic mutations. However, for many syndromes no mutation has yet been made visible at the molecular level. Indeed, as can be seen from the citation above, even in a syndrome where the mutation at the genetic level has been made visible, the pathway from the mutation to clinical picture is still 'unclear' – 'It is unclear how changes (mutations) in the DNA structure of the gene lead to the clinical findings'.

Syndromes such as Coffin-Lowry were mapped to chromosomes and to what is called a 'single gene'. The basis of this syndrome thus concerns what is rapidly beginning to look like old knowledge – in the wake of post-genomic understanding the genetic component of syndromes begins to look more complex. While 'genomics encompasses everything from sequencing genomes, ascribing functions to genes, and studying the structure of genes (gene architecture)', post-genomics 'takes these techniques further', to be able to study a person's 'entire genome' (Coleman 2006). But as will be seen, the genetic needs more than this – it needs more than individuals, it needs families. For example, the Coffin-Lowry foundation (including its website) is what Callon and Rabeharisoa (2008) describe as an emergent concerned group, a new social formation that is in part a response to the uncertainties of genetic diagnosis, in which associations of families, technoscience and the clinic can be seen to co-produce Coffin-Lowry as a genetic condition and as a pressure group. But what I want also to point to is how 'Coffin-Lowry' as a network of associations is also helping to produce and circulate the conception of syndromes as a new kind of clinical entity but one that still has so much that is undecided about it.

As is discussed later, particularly in Chapter 7, genetic medicine is one of the sites in which the shift – from single genes to genotype, from individuals to families, from diseases to syndromes – is being executed. This is because it is in the clinic that an (aberrant) genotype is being made visible as having its own clinical picture, not one simply located in the body of an individual, such as James Illa, but across the bodies of people who are biologically related, that is families.

For the moment, I want to stress how this science is embryonic and busy shrinking the field of the so-called normal. As the clinician in the above extract from the study says 'everyone has a syndrome' and, while many syndromes may not be as distinct as the picture of James Illa suggests, it is hard to see how many who currently think of themselves as normal will escape the net being created by dysmorphology as each genotype is made visible as having its own clinical picture.

A revival of medical dominance?

For these reasons, among others, I think dysmorphology offers a contemporary example of how medicine appears to be reviving its power in the wake of genetic discoveries in biology. Specifically, dysmorphology deploys methods of genetic profiling, such as genetic technoscientific discourse and technology, as well as discourses of embryology and human development, and draws all these together into its classic clinical methods for making pathology visible. But pathology here is at the level of the genes.

In terms of what I have called the first interface – the laboratory and the clinic – dysmorphology thus provides medicine with new as well as old alignments and new as well as old extensions. Through these alignments and extensions, medicine gains more grounds as a system of explanation, not less, including a place at the new frontier of genetic science. In addition, as a social institution – the interface between the clinic and the family – it gains even greater access to persons and families, becoming the managers of procreation strategies aimed at putting a stop on the reproduction of the abnormal and the proliferation of chronic disabling illness.

Ironically, then, my thesis of a percipient revival in medical power depends less on any process of natural selection and evolution. While the species of discourse we call medicine shows itself to be extraordinary at adapting to survive whatever a hostile environment throws at it, I am not suggesting it does so through some kind of Darwinian process of mutation. Nor do I suggest that medical dominance is accomplished through any essential or inherent fitness.

As I discuss in the next chapter, medical dominance is accomplished through medicine aligning itself with other institutions in ways that lead to its own engrossment in society. This is not to suggest that this process of engrossment is necessary or automatic. There is much hard graft involved in appropriating practices and discourses that can carry and move the social.

Nor does this graft just include simple processes of medicalization, or a colonization of other systems or of the life world. Similarly, dominance cannot be accomplished solely through practices of exclusion, although both medicalization and processes of exclusion do figure in my story. But it does depend upon *moments* of exclusion, moments when other systems, other grounds of explanation or possibilities for interpretation and conduct, get squeezed out.

My argument is that what is happening constitutes not only a medicalization of the biosciences, but sees the emergence of a new gaze (Foucault 2003b), a 'way of seeing' that is helping to constitute the genetic as a domain of explanation for the (mis)shaping and (de)forming of bodies, and the pathologies that flow from these deformations. In its focus on defining the misshapen, and the deformed, dysmorphology performs itself as a space of differentiation: as having a gaze that can distinguish between *different* aetiologies for pathologies in growth and form, even those molecular entities, the genotype, that are as yet invisible to laboratory science.

At the same time the clinic creates a space of deferral that legitimates the need for a future of more science and more technology. So let me say ahead I am not going to suggest that simply because medicine appears to involve an archaeology of different discourses, and a genealogy of multiple explanatory frameworks, that it represents a loss of purity; it has always been so. In the chapters that follow I show how in the clinic geneticists attach and detach themselves both to and from the knowledge offered by other scientific and technical domains of knowledge.

As I say, this is nothing new – medicine has always aligned itself with other scientific and technical domains. Social medicine and public health, for example, developed out of the alignment of clinical medicine, methods of population statistical analyses and engineering in the form of mains water and sewage works (Webster 1996). But what is of interest here is how clinical medicine is working its relations with the domain of an emerging and developing genetic technoscience.

Engaging with dogmatic ideas about the purity of domains (Latour 1993) is to misunderstand the relation between knowledge and power. So the study that follows abandons any notion that there is a purely clinical medical domain, or the dream of a purely laboratory-based science of genetics. Indeed, as will be seen, the laboratory of genetic science is distributed across many moments, occasions and locations, *including the interactions between the clinic and the family* – the very site in which medicine commands most power.

In this way the book explores the relation between medicine and genetic science in their co-constitution of the genetic as an emergent domain of culture and explanation. In particular it illuminates what this co-constitutive relation between clinical medicine and genetic science affords each in terms of authority, legitimacy and power.

An outline of the chapters

There are four parts to the book. The first part, 'Introduction and Background', Chapters 1 and 2, offers an introduction and gives valuable background to the book's three main themes. Chapter 2 sets out the four perspectives on medical power and elaborates on why the interaction of the gene and the clinic may be pivotal to my theme of a revival in medical dominance. While this chapter is critical to understanding the themes of the book, some readers might prefer to turn back to this chapter later in order to see first how contemporary doctors are performing genetic science.

In the second part of the book, 'The Gene and Medicine', Chapter 3 reviews the relationship between medicine and science, illustrating how this relation is performed in genetic medicine generally and by dysmorphology in particular. Chapter 4 describes how the relation between the laboratory and the clinic is specifically being constituted in genetic medicine as one of translation and co-construction in discovery, knowledge and innovation in genetic science. Chapter 5 shows how medicine in dysmorphology appears to not just be contributing to new understandings of genetic disease but to the relationship between genes and the growth and form of human beings.

In Part 3, 'Visualizing the Clinic', Chapter 6 takes us inside the clinic as an immersion in the real worlds of fleshy bodies, families and persons to show how dysmorphology creates its clinical pictures of syndromes. Chapter 7 presses how the clinic through its immersion in the family differentiates genetic from non-genetic disorders so that the clinic emerges as a kind of laboratory. In this 'clinic/laboratory' it is doubt and deferral that are as important as decisions and disposal, while the actual laboratory is relegated to the mundane production of tests and reports. Chapter 8 examines the visual culture of dysmorphology to suggest that it constitutes a new form of medical portraiture. What becomes visible in how dysmorphology constructs its portraits is the genotype–phenotype relation, a relation that cannot yet be revealed by technoscience alone. Thus I suggest that the clinic in dysmorphology is helping to provide a space of crossing for the ambiguous and elusive relation between the codes and digits of molecular biology and the substance of fleshy bodies: that is between *information*, *deformation* and *formation*.

In the fourth part of the book, 'The Family and Identities', Chapter 9 explores how the alignment of the gene and the clinic reconstructs the relation between bodies, persons and the human. It explores contemporary debates around how the recombinant biopolitics of the new genetics is eroding the very notion of the human. In this chapter, I show how there would be no point in a gene medicine that was only concerned with persons as biologically determined: gene medicine would have no power if it did not also reaffirm the human as of a higher order than mere substance. Specifically, paediatric genetic medicine, in all its crossings, reperforms the clinic as at the 'pinnacle' of the specifically human (Foucault 2003b), not the biological, or newly fashioned, 'life' sciences.

Chapter 10 revisits the relationship between medicine and the family, particularly in the context of contemporary discourses that institute parenting as an extension of actor-networks of public health. I show how the bodies of children become the visible manifestation and measure of good parenting, both in terms of looking good, being good and being healthy. However I also show how good parenting in these discourses is directed at lifestyle choice. I then go on to explore what family becomes in the genetics clinic and how at the same time as clinical processes intensify the responsibalization of parents as reproducing the future of healthy progeny, the alignment of the genetic clinic and the family institutes parents not merely as agents providing the right kind of environment for their child, but as family members whose biological matter may or may not need reforming.

Chapter 11 examines consultations in the clinic with the family, described by dysmorphologists as 'genetic counselling', a twin process of differential diagnosis and the calculation of risk of recurrence in other pregnancies. Focussing on interactions between families and clinicians, I show that family members are not so much disciplined in these encounters but are enrolled in the everyday work of clinical differentiation. I examine the nature and extent of this participation to show how they constitute relations of exchange, in which family members gift the clinic access to the family, both virtual and literal, in the form of bodies, photographs, histories and accounts, while parents are given a perspective, a way to knowledge that gives hope of a future of classification for what is wrong with their child/family. Specifically, family members are not simply informed about 'what is', rather, the clinic becomes a site of gathering, which engages parents in the epistemological work of objectification and differentiation, through which what is abnormal about their child is defined alongside clinicians' performance of deferral. The chapter shows how participation in this motility of clinical work moves parents between definition and deferral to excite consciousness of the riskiness of reproduction, elicit moments of reflexivity and accomplish shifts in perspective.

In the final part of the book, 'Conclusions', Chapter 12 summarizes the preceding chapters and returns to my initial argument of how medicine's dominant place is being reinvigorated by its alignment of the clinic, the gene and the family. I review theories of the erosion of medical dominance, including the geneticization of medicine. I show how in aligning the clinic and the new genetics, medicine is not simply being enrolled in a project coming from science but is itself complicit in the emergence of the genetic as a new domain that is engrossing medicine, science, social science and the social body. I conclude the book by summarizing my argument and offering a new way of thinking about medicine and power. I stress how the clinic is a site of bridging, crossing and gathering, between irreducible yet partially connected domains: the molar and the molecular, the flesh and informational codes, the social and the biological, the phenotype and the genotype, the individual and the family. I emphasise that it is in its switches in extension with other domains, in its intermittent and temporary attachments and detachments, to genetic technoscience one moment, to the clinic the next, and to the family the next, that medicine reinvigorates its power. I argue that commentators who augur the erosion of medicine completely underestimate its place as an institution whose authority is reinvigorated by its partial connection to science, and its partial connection to the family, and its partial connection to capital, and its partial connection to governing, and its partial connection to family and persons. Here I reiterate how we are in the midst of a return to a very functional approach to knowledge, rooted in ideas of need and impact, through which we are experiencing an intense medicalization of the biosciences. I then return to my theme of medicine's humanism, and the kinds of human being enacted in the clinic, to end the book with some thoughts on all the forms of life, ways of being and becoming, and the relationalities that the reinvigoration of the particular form of humanism in genetic medicine cuts out.

2 The clinic as the site of science

The signs and symptoms of disease do something more than signify the functioning of our bodies: they also signify critically sensitive and contradictory components of our culture and social relations. Yet, in our standard medical practices this social 'language' emanating from our bodies is manipulated by concealing it within the realm of biological signs.

(Taussig 1980, abstract)

Introduction

The previous chapter discussed how the path taken by the new genetics may be greatly affected by whether or not medicine retains its dominance in society. Ahead of explaining how the clinic is key to science, this chapter examines explanations for the rise of medical dominance and points out how it is classification – and its production of categories – that makes medicine both scientific and socially relevant.

The idea of medical dominance has long been debated in sociology and other fields. The thesis is based on an idea that there is a 'medical model', which in turn explains illness as a biophysiological phenomenon. Gabe *et al.* (2004) summarize the medical model thus:

> The medical model refers to the conception of disease established in the late nineteenth and early twentieth centuries, based on an anatomo-pathological view of the individual body.
>
> (p.125)

Often referred to as 'Western medicine', modern medicine emerged from the 'new sciences' of the 18th and 19th centuries and, subsequently, its associated group of clinical practices grew to dominate the treatment of illness in all the more developed nations.

According to Gabe *et al.*, this medical model: a) incorporated the *multiple paradigms* in the 18th century for diseases and their causes; b) developed *pathological anatomy* in the mid-19th century to locate specific diseases in particular organs or tissues; and c) demonstrated through *bacteriology* at the end of the

19th century that microbes cause major infections, such as tuberculosis and cholera. Together these culminated and coalesced around the clinical practice of making a correct identification of any pathology, or 'clinical diagnosis'.

As Gabe *et al.* suggest, clinical consultations increasingly focussed on the individual bodies of patients 'to the neglect of the wider social context' and they identify three core assumptions that established pathology within the corporality of the body: 1) that each disease has one cause for each disease (aetiology); 2) that diseases cause lesions in anatomy and physiology of the body – later to be broken down further into mechanisms of development (pathogenesis) and the structural alterations of cells (morphologic changes); and 3) that these processes underlie the 'signs' observed on the body and the patient's presentation of 'symptoms' (clinical manifestations).

For all this focus on the individual body, it is the search for accurate *diagnosis*, rather than the cures themselves, that becomes the crucial part of the 'physician's craft' and enables medicine to shape and influence society much more generally. For instance, the kind of identity work mentioned in Chapter 1 about who we are, and what life we might expect to enjoy, becomes increasingly entangled with this propensity for clinicians to offer a diagnosis. Similarly it is its ability to classify diseases, rather than cure persons, that allows medicine to act as the gatekeeper to many conceptual as well as material social goods. This is a role that, in turn, deepens its alignments with forms of governing on the one hand, and political economies on the other.

The fact that medicine also then became omniscient as a social institution (despite its apparent neglect of what Gabe *et al.* term the social context) calls for further explanation, and four perspectives can be delineated as the mainstays to this wider understanding of medical dominance: the sick role (Parsons), professional dominance (Freidson), medicalization (Foucault, Illich and Zola), and biopolitics, including processes of normalization (Foucault). These perspectives not only help elaborate the view that medicine has become the leading profession in terms of both status and monetary rewards; they also help explain how medicine became the most important functional organization through its focus on healing and repairing bodies. The upshot is that medicine acts as a dominant system of thought throughout society, as well as being a key social institution in its own right.

In the next four sections I explicate this wider thesis of medical dominance, taking in turn each perspective: the sick role, professional dominance, medicalization, and biopolitics. I do so partly to illuminate the importance of the clinic in linking medicine to society, but I also do so in order to challenge the current big story, mentioned in Chapter 1, that we are seeing a decline in medical dominance (for example, Rose 2007a, 2007b). I also want to address the corollary idea that we are witnessing the 'death of the clinic' (Rabinow 1992 drawing on Haraway; see also Latimer *et al.* 2006). As the later chapters unfold, it will become clear why I believe both these stories to be profoundly mistaken.

In the second half of this chapter, I go back through two of the perspectives of medical dominance, namely medicalization and biopolitics, to unpick more carefully the key contribution of the clinic. My aim here is to examine closely how it is that clinical practices radiate out into society and so affect its wider governance and culture. As I show, much of the prognosis about a decline in medical power lies in a poor understanding of how the clinic remains pivotal to medicine's own status of being scientific in its methods and procedures. Once this is better understood, it will become clear not only how the clinic acts as the cornerstone of the biological sciences' impact on society, but also why work in the clinic is proving key to developments in the new genetics.

Medicine and the sick role

There is a long history of theories that seek to explain how medicine came to be so dominant, and so align itself powerfully with other institutions. In particular Talcott Parsons, one of the major figures of mid-20th century sociology, argued that medicine occupied an important place in the social system. His idea of a social system was based on the premise that every subject, and every institution, had a 'part' to play that articulated with the whole.

This holistic theory presumed that there was a social contract of rights and obligations between individuals (the parts) and society (the whole), and, in his conception of the sick role, Parsons (1951) is offering a way of understanding how society and its parts act when the individual is unable to fulfil their usual duties and obligations:

> ... illness is a state of disturbance in the 'normal' functioning of the total human individual, including both the state of the organism as a biological system and of his personal and social adjustments. It is thus partly biologically and partly socially defined. Participation in the social system is always potentially relevant to the state of illness, to its aetiology and to the conditions of successful therapy, as well as to other things.
>
> (Parsons 1964, p.431)

Medicine's status as a social institution thus flows, according to Parsons, not simply from its power to cure the sick, but rather from its having the authority to *differentiate*. In the case of the sick role clinical differentation distinguishes between deviation from normal roles, obligations and duties that are legitimate on the one hand and illegitimate deviations due to time wasting and irresponsibility on the other:

> ... for common sense there may be some question of whether 'being sick' constitutes a social role at all – isn't it simply a state of fact, a 'condition'? ... Things are not quite so simple as that. The test is the existence of a set of institutionalised expectations and the corresponding sentiments and sanctions.
>
> (Parsons 1991, p.293)

In this model, as many commentators have pointed out, patients have to pass as legitimately sick: that is their troubles have to be made visible by a doctor both as *clinically pathological* and as a *disease*. Entry to the sick role had to be taken as temporary and doctors were accorded the right to physically examine patients' bodies and to inquire into intimate areas of their personal and physical life. In time doctors came to be used by other institutions, government, companies, schools, hospitals and even family, to help them to distinguish people faking it from the genuine thing: the hyperchondriacal, the hysterical and the malingerers from people with *real* illness.

In acting as 'gatekeepers', doctors were increasingly guided by rules of professional practice. The obligations and duties of the doctor, as a professional, were to apply a high degree of skill and knowledge to this problem of illness, to act for the welfare of the patient and the community, rather than self-interest or a desire for money or advancement. In return, doctors were granted considerable autonomy in their professional practice and placed in a position of authority in relation to patients. Consequently, as well as having a desire to get well, patients had to comply with 'doctor's orders'. This encouraged a growing passivity within the populace in the face of medical authority.

While failure to perform normal duties threatens the smooth working of other social institutions, such as the workplace or the family, to be sick enjoys a certain status. It is itself a social category: a state of being that occupies a '*structural*' position (Turner 1967). This is evident in the issuing of 'sick notes' to those deemed by doctors to be ill enough to gain all the rights and privileges of the sick person. It is also what Seale *et al.* (2001) call a 'blameless category'. It absolves the sick person temporarily from blame. To be sick is distinct from a general class of behaviour that would otherwise be seen as deviant or morally reprehensible (e.g. not going to work).

Medicine is thus much more than an important social institution in its own right. In Parsons' analysis, doctors appear as both the moral guardians of society and as gatekeepers to sickness as a role (and a blameless category provided certain conditions are met). Nonetheless, within this relation, sickness still has to be temporary. Problems arise for both the smooth running of medicine and for society when the temporality of sickness shifts to predominately chronic conditions. However, I still want to stress how, in this analysis, medicine is instituted as a site of *differentiation* – in this case differentiating the really ill from the rest.

Medicine as professional dominance

In contrast to Parsons, Eliot Freidson (1988) argues medicine is not so much a working institution that fits functionally into society, as it is a social institution that becomes self-interested in its own right. He shows how medical dominance depends for its power not upon a system of rights, duties and obligations, but upon *professional dominance* as a process of territorialization, monopolization and exclusion. Over time this dominance has sedimented the medical profession's status in ways that grant it not only control over its own work, but dominion over the work of other health workers, as well as over health resource allocation, health policy and the way hospitals are run.

Within this view medical dominance is accomplished through a relationship between the medical profession and the state. Specifically, the medical profession is on the one hand characterized by its autonomy from the state; for instance it defines its own ethical codes of practice and sets its own entry requirements to its various disciplines. On the other hand, it owes its exalted station within the social system to the licence that grants it authority to define and legitimate – including such matters as life and death, sickness and health (Freidson 1988).

More expansively, Irving Zola (1972) and Ivan Illich (1976) press the idea of medicine's authority in terms of how it has come to dominate people's ways of thinking: of how it works at the cultural level. Each questions the extent to which the medical model does not just influence, but takes over our ways of imagining what is normal. Their concern is over how medicine begins to shape identities, particularly in terms of what are appropriate ways of being and doing:

> ... medicine is becoming a major institution of social control, nudging aside if not incorporating the traditional institutions of religion and law. It is becoming the new repository of truth, the place where absolute and often final judgements are made, not in the name of virtue or legitimacy, but in the name of health. Moreover, this is not occurring through the political power physicians hold or can influence, but is largely an insidious and undramatic phenomenon accomplished by 'medicalizing' much of daily living, by making medicine and the labels 'healthy' and 'ill' *relevant* to an ever increasing part of human existence.
>
> (Zola 1972, p.487, emphasis added)

For Zola, medicine as an institution produces, and reproduces, culturally dominant ideas of normality and colonizes domains of existence that would come more appropriately under the authority of other institutions. As the repository of truth, Zola is suggesting that medicine has a normative function: in which final judgements are made about people in terms of their health. Thus Zola begins to draw out the relation between medicine and practices of normalization, in which people can be marked as healthy or ill.

Illich (1976), in the context of industrial forms of organization that create ill health, further emphasizes how medicine changes how we think about ourselves and what we do. Medicalization, Illich suggests, is achieved by 'social iatrogenesis', the process by which:

> [M]edical practice sponsors sickness by reinforcing a morbid society that encourages people to become consumers of curative, preventive, industrial and environmental medicine.
>
> (p.42)

Critically, for Illich this dependency on medicine is self-serving for the medical profession and its allies, such as the pharmaceutical industry. Indeed, as it deskills people, a kind of cultural iatrogenesis ensues, which destroys 'healthy responses to suffering, impairment and death' (1976, p.42), thus creating more ill health and a vicious circle in the need for more medicine.

More recent theories of medical dominance also stress how medicine is implicated in dividing practices through which the normal and the abnormal (as well as notions of the natural and the unnatural) are produced and reproduced (see for example, Fraser and Greco 2005; Lambert and Macdonald 2009). Yet for all that these theories expand our awareness of medical dominance, what they do not explain is how the medical model has become so insidious to everyday life.

Medicalization and the medical gaze

In discussing the theme of medicalization, I want to stress how the clinic is a site in which medicine *figures itself* as increasingly associated with the scientific method in the pursuit of truth. This is important, since it is this association that gives medicine its authority and institutes the clinic as the key site of discovery of truths about the body and about disease.

Michel Foucault is a French philosopher whose wide-ranging studies of key institutions, including the prison, the asylum and the hospital, have been much discussed in recent years. As he suggests in *The Birth of the Clinic* (2003a), it is in medicine associating itself with empiricism, and the supremacy of perception, that it both exercises its power and enables its practitioners to perform as sovereign subjects able to develop their methods and ways of seeing that, in turn, help constitute medicine as a form of positive knowledge.

In this way the hospital and the bedside are transformed into spaces of observation. However, Foucault is not describing medical perception as something that simply happens, as if 'seeing' was a process of direct unimpeded sight. To the contrary, the importance of his archaeological work on medical discourse through the ages is to show us that medical perception is an effect of a *discursive formation*. Specifically, Foucault traces and analyses modern medicine's *accounts of itself* as a new discursive formation, one that radically distinguishes itself from its past.

What Foucault sees as being argued in modern medicine's writings about itself is the possibility of medicine becoming a pure 'gaze', uncluttered by theory or superstition. Critically, though, what is 'seen' is not being held out to be a representation, an interpretation of what lies beneath the eye. Instead, modern medicine grants its doctors direct sight and experience of the real. The gaze is figured as a way to truth because of its distancing objectivity – accomplishing what Haraway (1991) calls the 'godtrick' – a detached objectivity that can read the book of nature. And, furthermore, it does this through the passive voice, in which any implication of their own agency is silenced (Birke 1998).

The perfection is what Foucault terms a 'disciplined gaze', a syncretic mix of interpretation and observation in which 'seeing' becomes 'saying' and 'saying' becomes 'seeing'. The 'gaze' as intricately conjoined modes of perception and annunciation makes the invisible visible (cf. Long 1992). Seeing, experience and knowing are different stages – but once it is part of the disciplinary gaze, *seeing* must then be pure. In Foucault's analysis, seeing is actually saying; and thus for medical perception to be able to see *the real* is a matter of semantics.

Foucault's point is that the medical gaze, medical perception, medical judgement, and clinical discretion are a part of the realities that speak and enact them. However, within modern medicine's framing of experience, discovering the truth can only be arrived at through direct perception of the real – as if this were possible prior to any 'map making'. So here we have the expression of the capacity of the gaze as being able to see the real: no longer a mere representation of the real.

Drawing on his ethnography of medical training at Harvard medical school, Byron Good (1997) captures something of this epistemological–ontological relation in his study of medicine and rationality. He states that, 'medicine formulates the human body and disease in a *culturally distinctive fashion*' (p.65), and explains:

> Doctors of course come to some extent to embody these formulations ... learning medicine is about learning quite fundamental practices through which medical practitioners engage and formulate reality in a specifically medical way. These include specialised ways of 'seeing', 'writing' and 'speaking'
>
> (p.71)

The message is clear: only by neophyte doctors following this path to knowledge can new knowledge of the body, and the truth about disease, be discovered.

For all this, the gaze does not simply discover facts and make disease visible. Rather, its expression is constitutive: both of *the objects of which it speaks*, and critically, for my purposes here, *of itself*. Here I am borrowing a notion of performativity from Michel Callon (2006) who states, 'a discourse is indeed performative if it contributes to the construction of the reality that it describes' (p.8). I explore this issue of what medicine is performing through its discourses further in the next section.

Medicine as biopolitics

While the performance of the medical gaze as scientific gives medicine its respectability, it is medicine's other associations that afford its more intense processes of medicalizing society. In his later work, Foucault is more particularly concerned with the relationship between science (including medicine) and forms of governing, than with the relations between medicine and science. Specifically, what he helps us to see is that medicine is deeply involved in the growth of the institutions that make up liberal forms of government, such as the hospital, the asylum, social medicine and public health (2000a, 2000b).

Within this perspective the hospital is not simply to be conflated with the clinic: rather it is a site that is an effect of relations between medicine, the clinic and the state, including the panoptic apparatus of surveillance and the survey. For example, with the emergence of public health in the 20th century as an alignment of medicine and public policy, there is extension of the medical gaze to the population and of the topology of medicalization to the home and the city: for instance through the apparatus that Armstrong (1983b) describes as the dispensary. This alignment of public health, policy and medicine is experienced in such technologies as immunization and screening programmes.

Foucault argues that the emergence of medicalization appears with the shift to capitalism, but that, ironically, medicine remains social in orientation because it includes the association of policy with the legitimation of the management of the health of populations:

> For capitalist society, it was biopolitics, the biological, the somatic, the corporeal, that mattered more than anything else. The body is a biopolitical reality: medicine is a biopolitical strategy.
>
> (Foucault 2000b, p.137)

Indeed for Foucault there are three strands that need to be considered in understanding what he calls the 'take off' of medicine at the end of the 18th century, composed of the development of a medical model and medical system (Foucault 2000b, p.134). These are: 1) biohistory – the 'effects of medical interventions at the biological level' (p.134); 2) medicalization – 'that is the fact that starting in the eighteenth century human existence, human behaviours, and the human body were brought into an increasingly dense and important network of medicalization that allowed fewer and fewer things to escape' (p.135); and 3) the economy of health – 'that is, the integration and improvement of health, health services, and health consumption in the economic development of privileged countries' (p.135). Specifically, he argues that it is after World War II, and the subsequent articulation of welfare medicine, that medicine's institutionalization is complete (Foucault 2004).

In all this, the emphasis on bio-politics goes well beyond the spatiality and temporality of the medical gaze; including the individuation of body-persons, or the advent of the clinic and the hospital. It is about how government's access to persons is legitimated by medicine and its attachments, including but not exclusively to biology. As Foucault stresses, 'it is understandable that medicine should have had such importance in the constitution of the sciences of man – an importance that is not only methodological, but ontological, in that it concerns *man's being* as object of positive knowledge' (2003a, p.197).

Critically then, on the pretext of discovering how to prolong life and relieve suffering, medicine legitimates incorporating man's being as subject to forms of surveillance that run much wider than the medical gaze. For example, the birth of social medicine (or public health) is made possible through medicine's alignment of biomedical analysis of bodies and their parts, and statistical technologies in the constitution of populations (Curtis 2002; Foucault 2000a), and of a normalizing judgement bodied forth in surveillance technologies such as we find in child health (Bloor and McIntosh 1990; Purkis 2002, 2003), or pregnancy screening programmes (Ginsberg and Rapp 1991).

Armstrong (1983a) and Silverman (1987) have each emphasized extensions to the scope of the medical gaze to include more than the body, so that clinical work no longer simply abstracts the patient as a social being. On the contrary, Armstrong and Silverman stress the emergence of a 'discourse of the social' that gives medical practitioners access to more extensive grounds upon which to call patients to account, so that 'a science of the subject has merely extended the range and disciplinary power of the professional gaze' (Silverman 1987, p.202).

This extension of the medical gaze can be seen in many areas of clinical work, including general practice, care of the dying (May 1992), and geriatric medicine (Latimer 2000). It is a process that does not just balance multiple perspectives, but can 'extend medicine's gaze to all aspects of bodily, mental, and social existence' (Kaufman 1994, p.430). This helps us to understand how medicine has become an agent of what Zola termed social control.

Having covered these four strands of the thesis of medical dominance, I use the rest of this chapter to develop the key aspects which, for me, explicate more fully the nature and extent of medicine's dominance in society. Particularly, I want to go back over and underline firstly the specific way in which medicine works as a science, and then secondly the idea that it is a technology.

The clinic as science

Critically, it is the clinic, not the laboratory, which is the locale for the discovery of modern medical knowledge. In *The Birth of the Clinic* (2003a) Foucault shows us a medicine that not only draws on science, but performs its field as if this is itself *scientific*. To accomplish its own way of seeing truly, the emergent clinic performs its 'detachment' from the knowledge of everyday life and thereby enacts a displacement of the social as being 'outside' medicine.

It is this aspect of Foucault's study that I want to press, that what he calls the birth of the clinic is the emergence of a way of writing and performing medicine that lays down the foundations for the association between medicine and the epistemological–ontological relation, which has become so valued and dominant in Euro-American culture.

> A scientific practice, in Foucault's account, is a particular set of codified relations between a precisely constructed knower and a precisely constructed object, with strict rules which govern the formation of concepts. One of these was that 'science' had set itself up as the ultimate form of rational thought. With the Enlightenment, scientific reason became the privileged way of accessing truth. According to this view for knowledge to acquire value as 'truth', *it had to constantly strive to become 'scientific', to construct and organize concepts according to certain rigorous criteria of scientificity.*
>
> (O'Farrell 2007, emphasis added)

While O'Farrell goes on to note that for Foucault scientific knowledge is not inherently 'superior' or more 'true' than other forms of knowledge, it remains the case that a disciplined way of seeing is a way to positive knowledge about the body and disease.

In this perspective, medicine's power to dominate comes from its capacity to perform itself as *methodologically* scientific, through its medical texts, as well as its diagnostic practices such as the 'clinical history' and the 'clinical examination'. The 'diagram' (Hetherington (2011) drawing on Deleuze (1988)) for this practice is the clinic:

> Clinics not only enabled comparative observations of disease manifestation; even more importantly, they reorganized the procedures of knowing or what Foucault called enunciative functions. Clinics were set up for the operation of the gaze, with patients lined up and laid out for inspection in a context understood to be the site of research and teaching as much as of the delivery of treatment. The individuality of cases became more important under the increased attentiveness and authority of the gaze, and clinics authorized the gaze and authorized the physician to ask to see, away from the social norms of domestic spaces. Out of this, new classifications emerged for organizing patients, medical knowledge, and authority. New possibilities of analogy and new relations of similarity and of relevance were developed. The subject positions of physician and patient were altered, with the individual physician gaining in authority. Disease as an object was reformulated, making possible the appearance of new theories of aetiology.
>
> (Alcoff, undated)

It is the clinic that becomes the key site for the production of truth about the human organism, and of disease, and, critically, it is here that new classifications began to emerge for organizing patients, medical knowledge and authority.

Additionally, as noted earlier, the clinic is where *the real* – not representations of the real – can be experienced and observed. Indeed, Foucault notes, drawing on Roucher-Derette (1807), that 'the observer reads nature … [h]e who experiments questions'. Consequently, the doctor has no use for the laboratory *as a part of the observation*:

> To this extent observation and experiment are opposed but not mutually exclusive. It is natural that observation should lead to experiment, provided that experiment should question only in the vocabulary and within the language proposed to it by things observed.
>
> (Foucault 2003a, p.131)

In this line of thinking, clinical truth not only precedes experimentation, it also *legitimates* it – providing the experimentation also derives from the same kind of direct observation that is integral to the 'disciplinary gaze'. To repeat, observation and experiment *are opposed but not mutually exclusive*: 'observation should lead to experiment, provided that experiment should question only in the vocabulary and within the language proposed to it by things observed' (Foucault 2003a, p.131).

As is discussed in Chapter 3, this means that laboratory science can never stand alone, but has to legitimate itself in terms of directing its work at clinically defined identities.

The clinic as a technology of governance

I now raise how the clinic's authority and power goes beyond its discursive performance of the medical gaze. Not only does the clinic become a site in which the non-relation/non-identity between the real and representation is acted out, there is a continuous acting out of a central paradox at the heart of Euro-American values: that the truth is to be found in the real. In all this I want to press something implicit to the source of medicine's power, matters that go back to the emphasis on medicine's categorical work in the introductory chapter.

The early knowledge produced by the clinic was used to create anatomical maps of the body and classificatory systems of disease and its effects on/in the body. These methods are now recognizable as the traditions of clinical nosography and the classificatory mentality of medical thinking (King 1982). Significantly, alongside this clinical work of observation and categorization, knowledge and method became standardized and codified. Thus the possibility arose for clinicians to be (re)presented not merely as natural scientists 'listening, deciphering, interpreting' but more grandly as sovereign subjects 'looking according to a grid of perceptions, and noting according to a code' (Foucault 1991, p.56). Crucially, alongside processes of objectification, the doctor as observer is both detached and has a fine, concrete sensibility (Foucault 2003a, p.148): the clinical moment is performed as a possibility of detachment and purity.

This said, it is also the building and fabrication for the 'medical model' as *a way of knowing* that constitutes particular realities (including the difference between the normal and the abnormal) for its diagnostic categories, and what is called 'the medical body' (Leder 1990). Through a correct and systematic reading of the body, signs and symptoms can be identified (or read), which are then 'recognized' as those of a particular diagnostic category (Atkinson 1997). Thus, exercised and disciplined in ways of seeing/saying, the gaze of the clinician becomes, via processes of sedimentation, a *technology*.

Within this view the doctor is both a disciplined *and* a sovereign subject. While any other member of the profession should be able to step up and say that they also see, in a process of affirmation, it is also open to each of them to say that they do *not*. Exactly how important it is for doctors in the clinic to be granted this power of discretion will be discussed throughout the rest of the book, but ahead of this it is worth making some preliminary explanation.

Powers of discretion

The methods of knowledge production developed in the clinic thus lie across two axes. The first axis allows the doctor-as-natural-scientist to move between their methods of classification, which read nature for signs, and their requisite technologies for making visible the inside of the body as the location of disease. The second axis allows the doctor to move between the naturalist observation of the causes and effects of disease on/in the body as modes of categorizing on the one hand, and classificatory systems that fix medical science as 'grids and codes' on the other.

Certainly medicine performs itself as the sole discipline that can read the book of nature on the body, especially whenever nature itself has gone adrift. For this to happen it is necessary for its practitioners to exercise their authority to make a diagnosis more or less in conformity to how any other well-trained clinician would. Each professional is expected to 'say' what there is to 'see'.

As Barnes (1988) explains, Weberian *powers of authority* rely on authorities being exercised along pre-set lines of delegation – rather like the way an electrical 'relay' conducts power along its circuits (see also Clegg 1989). Conjointly, however, medicine sees itself as granting its practitioners significant *powers of discretion* (Barnes 1988; Munro 1999a). Not only do doctors have the authority to say what they see, as 'sovereign subjects' (Foucault 1994), they also have the power to say they 'do not see' what others before them have said. Diagnostic classification appears at one moment stabilized (Bowker and Star 2000) by doctors acquiring a 'disciplinary gaze'; and at the next as needing remedial bolstering up by virtue of the discretion exerted by the doctor as sovereign subject.

Medicine, then, is a science that lies not just between deduction and induction. It also constantly requires both *the real as supplement*, and *the erasure of the real* to be credible. This is the nature of medical classification. To go back to the Introduction, and my discussion of the pathological, the red and itchy rash on the arm held out for clinical inspection is simultaneously real and yet its reality is erased wherever its significance as *clinical* is put in doubt by its not being 'seen', that is recognised, as the sign of a pathology.

It is in this interstitial space, between the real as supplement and its erasure, that clinical discretion can be found. The birth of modern medicine, that is *scientific medicine*, is thus simultaneously and paradoxically empirical and transcendent (Fuller 2007).

Ordering and reordering science

Reading Foucault helps us to see two important things. Firstly, that it is the association of the clinic with science ('scientific medicine') that gives medicine its authority. Secondly, Foucault's analysis also helps us to see how medicine does not act alone. This is to say that medicine becomes instituted as a 'centre of discretion' (Munro 1999a; Munro and Mouritsen 1996) through its associations with policy, and other discourses and technologies. This is in part why the alignment of the clinic and biological science can have such significant power effects in biopolitics.

In this chapter I have argued that medicine's power is partially an effect of its categorical work in the construction of diagnostic categories. Additionally, I have discussed how the clinic is instituted as a 'centre of discretion' in the naming and identification of the pathological. This is also key to medicine's power. As a centre of discretion, the clinic incorporates calculation in the creation of medical categories, but any calculation requires rooting in the real to differentiate the pathological. This is effected through the 'medical gaze', which can read the book of nature. I have particularly been stressing that it is when the clinic is pivotal to the scientific nature of medicine that medicine is so dominant.

Medical dominance relies, then, on its alignments with other bodies and discourses in networks of 'associations' (Callon 1986; Latour 1986), such as those with governments and markets, as well as with other disciplinary formations, such as engineering, religion or statistics, as described above. This much is clear.

In the remaining chapters, I go on to illustrate how the new genetics is being embedded into society – not through discoveries made in the laboratory as many expect, but rather through the identity work that is performed in the clinic. In this context, I show medicine as ordering and reordering the work of biological scientists on the one hand and the family and ideas of personhood on the other. This revival of medical power is illustrated in the rest of the book through a close examination of the embryonic discipline dysmorphology. As I go on to demonstrate, the dysmorphology clinic acts as a centre of discretion over the making of *genetic* clinical categories. Hence the ways in which the clinic works are infrastructural, not just to health services, but to new scientific enterprises.

Part II
The gene and medicine

3   Medicalizing science

Biology is destiny, the destiny of the individual and of the race ... This is a very real and immanent issue. If steps are not taken within a generation or two, disease and mental deficiency could very well run like wild fire through the entire species.

(Mathews 1999, p.222)

Introduction

The following three chapters examine the key relations between science and medicine. I trace how science has become increasingly beholden to medicine for its classification of needs, and how their relation is projected onto markets of the future in a reshaping of society. Throughout, I use the term 'the genetic' to encompass both medical *and* bioscientific knowledge and so build a perspective on the genetic as a socio-technical domain *in the making*.

Medicine and science co-constitute the genetic as a new domain of explanation about bodily effects, through their respective institutions – the clinic and laboratory. This perspective requires consideration of how relations between medicine and science get performed in the context of genetic medicine, and in this book I limit my focus to the production, consumption and disposal of evidence in dysmorphology as a branch of genetic medicine.

I want to stress that the field denominated by the genetic is emergent and unsettled and, further, that its flourishing and embedding in wider society, depends upon much more than discoveries in the biosciences or advances in molecular technologies. The more complex the genetic is in its influence on persons and disease, the better for both science and medicine. In this field we are not going to see the O-GOD approach to genetics popularized by the media (Conrad 1999): the very simplistic notion of genetics as the discovery of one gene, one disease. Rather, my point is to show how medicine's power is being re-established and reinvigorated through this opening up of the genetic as a new and complex frontier. Contrary to popular belief (e.g. Appleyard 2012), the more complex and problematic the frontier, the better for medicine!

My aim is to show how doctors in genetics perform themselves as helping to make the genetic happen. As such, they do not see themselves as merely 'applying' science. Specifically, what gets enacted by specialists in genetic medicine, and by dysmorphologists in particular, is a special medical gaze that affords the recognition and description of naturally occurring (as opposed to experimentally produced) forms of life that, in turn, imply a problem with their biological development. This work typically involves looking for, and investigating, the visible expression of aberrations at the genetic level. As I have already indicated, these clinical geneticists claim to be helping to shape the science of growth and form. They are participating in the mapping of the genetic in relation to human development, one of the most fundamental areas of the biosciences – the other two being reproduction and ageing.

Holding my exploration of how relations between the clinic and the laboratory are enacted in dysmorphology against contemporary debates on science and medicine, this chapter begins to build a picture of how dysmorphology is helping to reinvigorate the place of clinical medicine as a site for the production of knowledge, not just its consumption. It may well be the case that the clinic's hold on knowledge has been somewhat attenuated in recent years through its alignment with managerial and audit cultures (Armstrong 2002; Bury and Taylor 2008) but, as we see in the following chapters, pronouncements about the death of the clinic are certainly too hasty.

(Dis)locating dysmorphology: from backwater to metropolis

The study I undertook radiated out from the clinical genetics service of one major UK teaching hospital providing clinics across a large region of the British Isles. This regional medical genetic service was one of 12 in the UK (details of each service can be found by visiting Genetic Alliance UK at http://www.geneticalli-ance.org.uk/services.htm#WA). The services, which are part of the National Health Service, are free at the point of delivery, and are sites of university medical research and education, providing training and courses in genetic counselling.

The regional service that formed the focus of the current study includes experts, laboratories and genetic counsellors, some of which are located in the main department. Practitioners located in the main department also travel to other hospitals to hold clinics, while others are based in other hospitals. All members of the service communicate and meet regularly at clinical and academic meetings, discussing and sharing cases. Some members of the medical staff may be employed as NHS doctors, but are also university lecturers or professors. While most are engaged in research, some doctors are still learning to be clinical geneticists. This is reflected in the organization of medical genetics. Teams acting under a consultant are made up of specialist registrars, specialist nurses, trainees and so on and so forth.

At first sight, dysmorphology hardly looks like a discipline – for instance, there is no department of dysmorphology. In my first visits to the Medical Genetics Institute (the home of the regional service that was the starting point for my ethnography) it did not seem possible that my intuitions could be right. Located in a National Health Service teaching hospital, as it is called in the UK, the Medical Genetics Institute was difficult to find in the chaotic labyrinth of buildings and roads that make up the departments, laboratories, and medical school.

The Institute is housed in a small building about ten years old at the back of the main hospital, opposite the paediatric and obstetric unit. As a first impression it did not appear to be anything that was going to turn out to be a critical site. However, as things turned out, its location here signifies the first of dysmorphology's important relations – with paediatrics and reproductive medicine, and through them, to human development.

The entrance to the institute is in a sub-basement. The waiting room and the consulting room contain no clinical equipment. There is no bustle, and there are no beds, no white surfaces, no brash and bold machines – nor, indeed, any of the paraphernalia usually associated with the spectacle of modern medicine. Little to suggest, therefore, that there would be much reward in following around the consultants as a key part of my ethnography.

Here I meet two consultants in a small, dull interview room with boxes of toys, a few comfortable chairs and a coffee table. My impression is of a *medical backwater*. Everything reflects the story of the NHS in terminal decline: doing research and medicine on a shoestring. Later when I visit the main protagonist's office to plot the research design, I am shocked at just how tiny it is: partitioned off by glass at the back of an open plan office of secretaries, it consists of about 4 square metres of floor space. This space has no natural light and is largely taken up by a desk and two chairs, some filing cabinets, and a computer, with every available surface covered in files and papers. All this hardly seems compatible with the consultant's reputation as an eminent geneticist of international renown.

Later when I visited other consultants in their home institutes and departments some, like Dr White, were located in cubbyholes in dreary and old-fashioned hospital departments of medical genetics. Others, however, met me in the much more contemporary buildings of the Genetics Knowledge Parks, like those at Cambridge or Newcastle. While these parks are a part of university medical schools, they also represent a new site of medicine. For example, the one in Newcastle is in the 'International Centre for Life' (http://www.life.org.uk/), which opened in 2002, 'with funding of over £10M over five years, enabling the university to draw on its research strengths in the fields of cancer, ageing and human development' (http://www.ncl.ac.uk/1834/history/timeline/).

I am suggesting that this apparent range of investment, from cubbyholes in departments in teaching hospitals to these contemporary monuments, signifies something about the emergence of medical genetics at this time. Locating medical genetics in Gene Parks symbolizes the manufacture of a new culture of science and medicine around interdisciplinarity, closely tied to contemporary ideas about openness and innovation (Strathern 2004a, 2004b).

With the double helix displayed iconically in logos and sculptures (see Figure 3.1) like a homogenizing brand (Myers 1990), the scale of these contemporary architectural structures associates genetics with 'tech'. The alignment between tech, the genetic and medicine is constituted as positive, giving a message about the future, as well as promising economic and social value. Heralded as public spaces, epitomized by calling them parks or villages with events and exhibitions dedicated to education and public engagement, these sites associate an idea

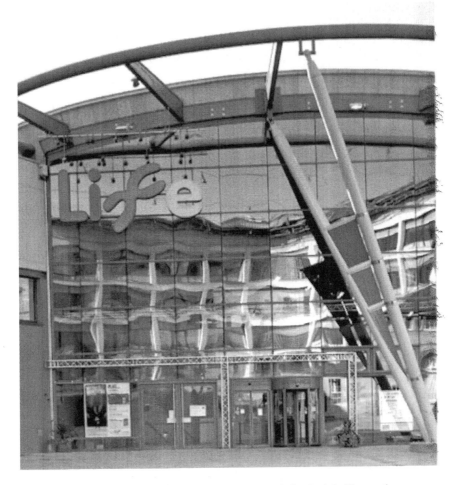

Figure 3.1 The iconic double helix and the Gene Knowledge Park in Newcastle.

of science and medicine with creativity, technology and innovation, rather than with sick bodies and minds, or the hospital or clinic (see also Strathern 2004b). In creating possibilities for interaction with science there is a sense that public engagement is being put at the heart of this new science culture.

What I take from this range of homes for medical genetics – and from the dysmorphologists who dwell there – is the sense that medical genetics during the first decade of the new millennium was a variable space of investment *and* competition for universities, medical schools and governments. Creating, as well as responding to, a growing 'market', medical genetics is located in an emerging political economy of science, health research and clinical practice. In the UK, it is positioned explicitly at an intersection between medical schools and the National Health Service. Increasingly in England the emphasis is on links between public and private finance motored by an impact discourse of the need to boost failing capitalist economies.

I should add that much of this massive investment has happened since my first visit in 2002 to my 'home' department, described earlier. Indeed, this institute also now has a new building, if nothing quite so grand as those to be found at Newcastle's Life Centre, or at the Cambridge Knowledge Park. The Institute is also associated with, rather than located in, a Genetics Knowledge Park. Such changes symbolize how much medical genetics has been a growth industry.

Critically, it is the technological spaces of the Genetics Knowledge Parks, rather than the Intensive Care Unit of the high tech hospital, which form the new 'spectacle' of medicine. They advertise, promote and magnify an investment in the idea that it is knowledge and science – far from the bedside of the sick – that can help cure the ills of modern societies: the cancers, the Alzheimer's, the ageing, and even, perhaps, the economic downturns. They constitute the new 'fronts' of medicine, seemingly forcing the clinic and the hospital, and even to some extent the laboratories, backstage.

Despite all this, as will be seen, the consultants still go to the backstage to do their clinical work. Each of the consultant geneticists I visited, no matter their location, were practising clinicians as well as publishing researchers.

Surprisingly, in the building up of their knowledge base and in the defining of their discipline and expertise, I show in what follows how much dysmorphologists rely on immersion in the clinic and the family. Like ethnographers, the scientists and clinical scientists each still need engagement with the 'mess', materialities and socialities of everyday life. However, there is more to be examined here in regard to how the relations between medicine and science are being performed by these new spaces, and I press this aspect next.

Engineering the 'good (healthy/wealthy) society'

The next aspect of medicine's relation to science to which I draw attention is connected to that other facet of medicine: its humanism and its place in European intellectual, social and political history. In addition to its key place in terms of biopolitics, discussed in Chapter 2, medicine has played an integral role, as Charles Webster (1996) asserts, in 'the formation of Western culture' (p.34).

Medicine's complex status as an institution is important here. This status, as both a site of scientific methodology and as important to intellectual, social and political history, helps constitute medicine as an obligatory passage of legitimation for governmental strategies as well as for science. As discussed in Chapter 2, Foucault claims this history is strongly associated in Europe with the relationship between welfare and capital: the idea that what is good for the individual is good for society *and* for capital. The underpinning ethic demands that the distribution of responsibility and resources has to be accounted for in terms of the meeting of *needs* (shifting between individual, societal and capital).

As indicated in my earlier discussion in Chapter 2, one amongst many technologies legitimated by medicine is *the experiment*. The key point here is that the need for experimentation requires legitimatizing, particularly in terms of funding experimental science. This legitimation does not come from the observation of causal relations, or from the development of hypotheses that require testing (and which may or may not have profound implications for the design of interventions). In a more functionalist world, the need for experimentation requires legitimation in terms of *social* need. Specifically, the material and embodied genealogy of science and medicine is intertwined.

Indeed, health and wealth have this long and entangled trajectory in the history of medicine and its alliance with governments. This is due to the association between the need for knowledge about the body and disease, and their relation to wealth and enhancement. It is worth remembering here that the clinic is only one of medicine's sites of operation: there are many others, for example the home, the family, government health and social policy, the law, and increasingly 'www//http'. While there is merit in the view that these operate as satellite sites orbiting around the production of knowledge radiating from the clinic, medicine appears and reappears intermittently across these sites as a 'distributed and multi-sited knowledge system', which includes ethical plateaus and civic political contests embedded in disputes over 'government health and social policy mantras' (Fischer 2005).

Medicine's place as a social institution, and its promotion of particular values and metaphysical ideas, is part of the translation of innovation into a force for good. This goes as far back as the alchemists' laboratories of the Medieval and Renaissance periods in Europe. While these laboratories had a practical function, their significance was also connected to wider metaphysical ideas: they were experimental sites associated with the making of the philosopher's stone – 'the magical substance for transforming base metals into gold and *indefinitely prolonging life*'[1]

> There is also an operative and practical alchemy, which teaches how to make precious metals and pigments, *and many other things better and more plentifully than they are made by nature.*
>
> (Bacon, emphasis added, cited in Pinkowski 2004, p.26)

Implicit in this is that the legitimation for laboratory work was seldom only functional or economic: its legitimation rested as much in the idea of its pursuit of a cure for morbidity and mortality, and, as such, in finding a way to *improve on nature*.

Re-medicalizing science

One of the most important sources of legitimation for science continues to be an idea of enhancement through the improvement of health. As Shapin (2000) raises the issue:

> That is one – blindingly obvious – reason why the ability to prevent and cure disease, to alleviate suffering and to extend human life has recurrently been

used as a public test of the truth and power of philosophic and scientific systems, and why the learned too might share in that public assessment.

(p.132)

Quite so. However, I want to invert Shapin's argument to suggest that, in the contemporary relation between the so-called basic biological and clinical sciences, we can see a *remedicalization* of science. It is not so much that the science today simply gets tested by its capacity to prevent and cure disease, or alleviate suffering. Rather, the life sciences are being called upon to develop and hone their foci and practices in relation to medically defined needs *in advance*.

What is being done inside what we call science – as though it were one hegemony of practices – has also to be examined for the translation of interests effected by these relations between medically defined needs and scientific practice and process. By committing to research programmes whose aims and objectives are to 'alleviate suffering and to extend human life', it is not merely productivity that is to grow. In the endless cycle of production, consumption and growth upon which capitalist economies depend for their survival, basic science is being translated and changed in its nature.

We must acknowledge here how scientific funding programmes and government strategies are increasingly engineering these domains – medicine and science – in order to intertwine their organization into close knit 'partnerships'. This is not just to note how medicine is being reorganized by new discoveries in science. Instead it is to understand how the biosciences are being reorganized in relation to this re-defining of needs; and that for their own survival, bioscientists need to demonstrate to their funders and to the wider public that they are addressing this agenda.

We can see these effects in contemporary funding requirements, which are setting research agendas. For example, in terms of funding, there is an 'agenda setting' (e.g. the European Research Council's agenda, or the strategic priorities of the major funding councils) through which the basic sciences are increasingly being called upon to legitimate their interests, foci and activities not in terms of the pursuit of knowledge, but of knowledge that will be useful in terms of improving health: they need to show how they help reveal correlations between biological processes and the development of disease or the sustaining of health, together with the direction of possible interventions. These relations are expressed in grandiose mission statements and visions, such as the statement of their vision on the UK's Biotechnology and Biological Sciences Research Council's (BBSRC, undated) website:

Our vision
    To lead world-class 21st century bioscience, promoting innovation and realising benefits for society within and beyond the UK.
    BBSRC has a unique and central place in supporting the UK's world-leading position in bioscience. We are an investor in research and training, with the aim of furthering scientific knowledge, to promote economic growth, wealth and job creation and to improve quality of life in the UK and beyond.

In the coming decades bioscience will be central to providing solutions to major challenges, such as:

- Feeding 9Bn people sustainably by 2050
- Developing renewable 'low carbon' sources of energy, transport fuels and chemicals to reduce dependence on dwindling oil reserves
- Staying healthier for longer as lifespan increase and society ages

Our vision is structured around **world-class bioscience**, **key strategic research priorities** and **enabling themes** – methods we will use to achieve our aims.

The BBSRC is the largest UK public funder of 'non-medical research', with an annual budget of around £445M, and we can see from their vision and strategy that some of the work they will fund has to demonstrate benefits and impact in terms of improving quality of life as well as being able to provide solutions that will help people 'stay healthier for longer'.

Now if the dominant discourse over what counts as health and quality of life is medical, then, increasingly, bioscience is going to become intertwined with medically defined needs and problems. For example, the BBSRC publish news about scientific breakthroughs. One of the categories here is 'Health News', and includes reports on how basic research has contributed to discoveries or interventions into specific diseases and their treatments such as bipolar disorders or Alzheimer's. The efficacy of bioscientific exploits in these kinds of funding programmes is thus increasingly being explicitly harnessed to market values, health, wealth, job creation and economic growth.

We can also see this intermingling in the organization of basic bioscience, medicine and innovation into new forms of 'Big Science' (Galison 1994) and the proliferation of 'interdisciplinary' scientific institutions described above – what Clarke *et al.* (2003) are describing as 'Biomedical Technoservice Complex, Inc'. For example, The Wellcome Trust's Sanger Institute whose mission makes explicit the relation to medically defined problems:

> At the Sanger Institute we aim to make a real contribution to global health, a responsibility that derives from our position as a world leader in genomic research. For example, we are carrying out large scale research programmes dedicated to investigating the biology and genomics of malaria, which kills over one million children in Africa each year and causes debilitating illness in over half a billion people worldwide. We also invest in research that elucidates the genetic basis of cancer and metabolic and cardiovascular disease, which are a significant part of the global health burden.
>
> (Wellcome Trust, undated)

Or the 1000 Genomes Program:

> An international research consortium has announced the 1000 Genomes Project, an ambitious effort to sequence the genomes of at least 1000 people

to create the most detailed and *medically useful* catalogue to date of human genetic variation.

(Wellcome Trust 2008, emphasis added)

Similarly, the National Science Foundation (NSF) in the US with an annual budget of about $6.9 billion in 2010, has a mission 'to advance the national health, prosperity, and welfare' (NSF 2010).

Somewhat controversially, Rose (2007b) asserts that medicine is not just being molecularized and technologized, but also *capitalized* in ways that demean it and erode its authority and power. There is, for instance, an increasing tie with Treasury-defined objectives that make explicit how the sciences are being enrolled in health improvements that will have specific economic/societal gains; and, in the US, concern over the potential 'domination of the nation's scholars by Federal employment, project allocations, and the power of money' (Shapin 2008, p.81).

Although he is making an important point, I think Rose is too sweeping in making his claim, for what is happening is not just a simple capitalization of medicine, or science. Rather, the relation between medicine and capital is nothing new. As Foucault's analysis of biohistory discussed in Chapter 2 helps us see, medicine's position in relation to capitalism has long been in terms of governing and shaping the social. Indeed, the position of medicine as 'in between' capital and health is well represented in a lovely engraving from the website Pandora's Box (undated), which explores relations between medicine and the humanities, arts and sciences. The engraving draws on ancient iconography, with Esculapius (Medicine) as a figure standing in between Mercury (Merchants) and the Graces (Medicine, Hygiene and Panacea). The caption reads as follows:

> Esculapius dealt with Patients – Merchants make deals with Clients Esculapius is linked with a Constellation of Idealistic Medical Ideas Mercury or Hermes is linked with Haemaphroditism and Mercantile Mercenary views.

Here, medicine is represented as in between the merchants on the one hand and the three graces on the other. As such, historically medicine is the link: the conduit between the two sides, capital and idealistic notions of health as a *metaphysical* good. I am suggesting that this relationship persists today.

This is not to insist that in the backstage of 'small science', boundary work between applied and basic science is not going on in the clinic. As I have shown above, these fronts can hide more than they reveal. But there are also accountability practices here through which branding science as being 'of use medically' putatively *adds value*. Indeed, in the earlier analysis of the medical gaze, we have already seen how the association between the clinic and science also adds value.

Medicine as adding value to the biosciences

In this chapter, I have been pressing how the proliferation of life science research may increasingly depend upon its medicalization. Specifically, how the legitimation and significance of research in genetics is being articulated in relation to health needs defined by medical discourse as for the good of society, including wealth and health. Indeed, after Verran (2011), this can be understood as an 'ontic politics', in which the utilitarian and the metaphysical, the ethical and the instrumental, value and values, become jointed together in the manufacturing and securing of technoscientific futures.

This particular alliance of science and medicine, and what I am calling the medicalization of the basic sciences, and their transmogrification into 'Life' sciences, can be seen as an effect of the parallel and intertwined agendas of making science more ethical and relevant, encapsulated in ELSI (Ethical, Legal and Social Implications) Programs throughout the Western world, whose aim is not just to get science into society but also to get society into science (Strathern 2004a).

Löwy (1996), probing the 'seemingly natural process of the genesis and development of medical facts' (p.19), stresses how the generation of medical facts legitimates the need for the pursuit of particular aspects of science. There are serious issues here. On the one hand, as Löwy goes on to suggest, medicine, as the site that to some extent determines the *need* for science and technology to enhance society in terms of health and wealth, does so at the expense of other possible ways of seeing a problem. On the other hand, in genetic medicine there is even more to the relation between medicine and science than the possible detection of, and intervention in, disease processes, including genetic abnormalities.

This brings us to the issue of flow and direction, and to how the definition and significance of effects become medicalized as diagnostic categories that need to be addressed by science in its association with medicine. The categories themselves are medical: cancer, malaria, diabetes, inflammatory disease, the myriad genetic disorders or syndromes; even ageing itself is increasingly being categorized in terms of disease.

These medical categories are being mobilized and enrolled to legitimate new forms of interdisciplinary 'science'. But they also represent assemblages, stabilized as solid medical diagnostic categories. Questions therefore arise as to how these assemblages, such as genetic diagnostic categories, come into being. I address this aspect by examining how the relation between science and medicine is accomplished within genetic medicine in the following three chapters.

Conclusion

In this chapter I have begun to suggest how an alignment with medicine acts as social and cultural capital (Bourdieu 1984) for bioscience, and vice versa. This is to say that an association with science does not just add value to medicine, as argued by Foucault and others and discussed in Chapter 2. More and more, medicine is going beyond adding value to science to imbue it, additionally and explicitly, with its values. The upshot is science having to address medical problems in order to give itself *moral* as well as economic purpose.

It is in this identification and definition of which problems need to be addressed, that the entangling of medicine and science is at its most potent. Here the renaming of the 'biosciences' as 'life sciences' is significant: connecting bioscience to 'life' and 'lives' makes explicit its association with objectives that address the need to improve quality of life and health. The interjection of medically defined objectives associates life science research with health, welfare and capital to joint both moral and economic agendas.

We can see in the medical fronts I have described in this chapter an engineering that reinforces the interdependency of science and medicine. This is not just to engineer societies in terms of the good life, the good society, but also in terms of the 'goods' of capital. While I have pointed out that this is nothing new, the life sciences in their association with medicine are meant to address the market, and figure more and more in the stimulation of wealth creation.

What I want to underline here, though, is how that which counts as science is itself being reshaped by a particularly insidious process of medicalization: a process that involves medicine's location as aligned with policy and government and an association with the need to generate knowledge that will help promote not just a healthy society but also a wealthy one. I am suggesting that, in the growing climate of functionalism, science is being associated with medicine in ways that do not just enhance medicine, but are actually medicalizing science – even to the point of eroding distinctions between basic and applied science. This is important since debates over the geneticization of medicine, as well as talk of the erosion of medical dominance, appear to miss this aspect of the interaction of science and medicine.

In the next chapter, as I get behind the fronts of science and medicine and go *inside* their intersection in dysmorphology, we can begin to see that the co-constitutive and interdependent relations between medicine and science also lay claim to shaping the science of *normal* human development.

4   The 'translation' of growth and form

> The key to understanding form is development; the process through which a single-cell egg gives rise to a complex, multi-billion-celled animal ... I have described the genetic toolkit for development and how its discovery was driven by the study of spectacular mutants that made the wrong number of body parts, or put a part in the wrong place, or lacked some major structure all together. Most of the time, thankfully, nature gets it right and flies and babies are born with the right number of parts in all the right places.
>
> (Carroll 2005, p.82)

Introduction

In the previous chapter I introduced the notion that, in the contemporary land-scape of politics, markets and research funding, relations between medicine and bioscience are being intensified, offering some evidence for how bioscience is being increasingly medicalized. In this chapter I problematize this fissure further by challenging ideas that dichotomize science from medicine into separate domains. Particularly questionable is the presumption that science is the major site of discovery and that medicine merely hosts the 'application' of science. Rather, what we are beginning to see is how the 'genetic toolkit' for development in humans is partly evolving from what Carroll, a molecular biologist, calls the clinical study of 'spectacular mutants that made the wrong number of body parts, or put a part in the wrong place, or lacked some major structure all together.'

Much current thinking treats medicine as a passive territory being colonized and transformed by innovations from science and technology. There is a central problem with this view. To separate science and medicine in this way is to under-stand the relations between them in terms of a diffusion model through which theoretical discoveries and innovations in 'science' are imagined as knowledge and innovation dripping down into practical activities such as 'medicine'. Some of this thinking is embedded in the differentiation between the clinic and the laboratory as different kinds of organizations: the latter concerned with discovery and innovation and the former with delivery and intervention. Indeed, diffusion models are also embedded in the policy and artefacts organizing clinical and applied science on the one hand and basic science on the other.

A more contemporary articulation of knowledge being radiated outwards is encapsulated in the idea of 'translational research'. For some this has the rather simplistic idea that: 'A translational scientist should be able to move an idea all the way from basic research to a clinical application and back to the lab to inform more basic science' (Broussard 2011). Others like Latour (1987), as will be discussed, are much more radical and sophisticated in their conception of translation.

This more radical view sees translation as a ubiquitous process that is endemic in all aspects of innovation and, consequently, eschews the notion of basic research as the single major source or origin for discovery, in which technological change is seen as a linear process (research > invention > development > innovation > diffusion):

> The linear view of technological change has recently been superseded by a non-linear conceptual model featuring feedback loops emanating from each stage (Kline and Rosenberg 1986). In this alternative model, basic science can fit into the process of innovation at any stage. *Moreover, the very idea of a source or an origin point of technology is misleading because innovation is an emergent, interactive activity.* It involves many actors who cooperate or oppose one another (Akrich, Callon and Latour 2002). Science and scientists ... are no exception.
>
> (Callon 2006, p.4, emphasis added)

Distinctions and divisions such as that between applied and basic science, useful as they may have once been in terms of boundary work, are also being eroded in the new political agendas and the organization of science funding. As discussed in the previous chapter, biosciences are increasingly gaining their legitimating discourses from their alignment with medicine – the rationale being to expand the prosperity of nations, as well as to help improve their health.

In line with Michel Callon's comments, quoted above, I am going on to show how discourses of genetic medicine present 'circuits' in which we move from practices to inscriptions and from inscriptions to practices in the constitution of new medical entities. But I want to go beyond simply showing how these discourses perform medicine as co-constitutive of medical entities, important as this matter is. So in the rest of the chapter, and in the chapter that follows, I pick up on Carroll's position cited above, and argue that dysmorphology in genetic medicine emerges – particularly in those discourses and practices relating to the natural history of syndromes – as claiming to help shape the science of growth and form.

The present chapter begins with a brief insight into the world of dysmorphology. This helps to illustrate how the relation between medicine and science is performed in dysmorphology. After a discussion of debates in the social sciences over the relations between the clinic and the laboratory, I then move between different discursive practices to show how the clinic in genetic medicine is very far from being reshaped by innovations coming from the laboratory. What emerges instead is a picture of the complex relation between science and medicine working through translation effects from invention and innovation back and forth between the clinic and the laboratory.

The theatre of dysmorphology

Imagine being in a large, bright and airy auditorium – very modern and generous with its padded seats sweeping down to a large front area (see Figure 4.2). There is an elevated podium on the left, a huge screen behind, and another large screen to the right. The theatre is completely full, some sit with notes and papers while others have laptops sitting in front of them. An energetic and forceful woman is standing to the side, about halfway up the aisle, directing the ceremony. It is all beech wood, steel and glass.

As the person at the podium talks, images are projected onto the large screen behind them as well as to the other screen to the side of them. These images show assemblages of photos of children and babies, details of parts of bodies, various diagrams, scans of brains, strange images of strings of small objects and so on and so forth. The images appear and disappear during the talk, giving a medical genetics' case history. This consists of a history of the pregnancy and birth of the child, a history of their growth and development since birth, details of any health problems, results of tests, and descriptions of the child and their family's body parts and behaviour. They usually also present a family history, represented on screen as a 'family tree', and what is sometimes referred to as a medical pedigree. On the other screen to the right, different lists of features are being projected while another person, a middle-aged man, is sitting at his desk, tapping away at his laptop just below the podium (just off the picture and to the right in Figure 4.2).

I am in the lecture theatre in the Wellcome Trust Building at the Institute of Child Health, University College, London. The woman is Professor Fox and, as my study progresses, I learn to think of her as one of the mothers of dysmorphology in the UK. The younger person at the podium reading from their notes is a neophyte geneticist. The man sitting at a computer in front and to the right of the podium is Professor Smart and I learn to think of him as the father of UK dysmorphology.

At a later interview, when I meet Professor Smart face to face, I find out he was scrolling through the dysmorphology database of features, searching for a match with what the younger doctor at the podium is reporting. During this later interview, Professor Smart shows me this database. He tells me that to be a dysmorphologist:

> You have to have a multiple choice sort of mind, like all the facts are there *but you don't just regurgitate them, somebody gives you options and you know what it is.* That's what I think anyway … And also you had to be good at visual recognition as well – which seems to be genetic.
>
> (Author interview, 2003–2004, emphasis added)

Good at visual recognition, indeed. For there are over three thousand syndromes described in this database, with each syndrome broken down into hundreds of

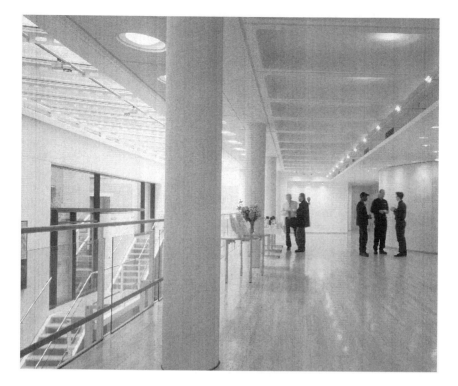

Figure 4.1 Atrium, Institute for Child Health, Wellcome Trust building, University College London. With kind permission of ORMS Architecture Design and Nick Kane http://www.nickkane.co.uk

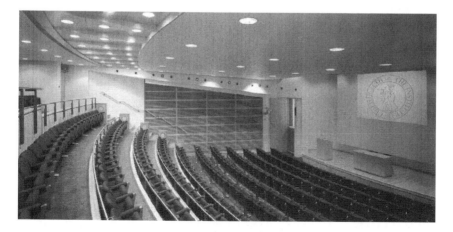

Figure 4.2 Lecture theatre, Institute for Child Health, Wellcome Trust building, University College London. With kind permission of ORMS Architecture Design and Chris Gascoigne http://www.chrisgascoigne.com

features, traits, and expected clinical findings, such as test results. But Professor Smart is also stressing how, in order to be a good dysmorphologist, you don't just regurgitate, you *know* what it is.

The particular occasion I am attending is a meeting of the London Dysmorphology Club (cf. http://www.clingensoc.org/Dysmo/index.htm), whose home is this new, quite beautiful building for the Institute of Child Health (see Figures 4.1 and 4.2), based at Great Ormond Street Hospital for Sick Children, a world-leading centre for paediatric medicine and research. This is the academic meeting of the UK network of expert dysmorphologists and trainee medical geneticists where the discipline is being established and passed on. The people in the audience are there to debate the presentations and, as I am finding out from Professor Smart's interview, to learn how to *do* dysmorphology. So the audience sits, listens and watches. They are seeing how he does his search. Indeed, a good number of those present in the audience also have computers and are scrolling down inside the same database as Professor Smart. They mimic him, enacting what he enacts, and they listen and watch the presenters as they relate the case history.

The assemblages of things on the screen represent the child, the family, and the parts of them that are possbile signifiers. As well as photographs of children, their distinguishing features, and their biological relations, they include laboratory results, images of chromosomes, scans and x-rays. The performance of the clinical gaze thus brings the laboratory and the family into association. On these occasions there is nothing about the family or the child that marks them as social beings: they are figured almost entirely in terms of their signs, symptoms, history and, of course, the visual images.

Sometimes the person at the podium is very pleased with himself or herself – they have a diagnosis. Often they have no diagnosis and Professor Fox engages the audience in 'guessing' what the diagnosis might be. There is a lot of audience interaction and participation, debate and questioning. What is being decided, in ways that go to the heart of Callon's view of translation, is what is abnormal and/ or unusual, about the child and/or other family members. Equally, what is also being decided, often explicitly, is what is normal or usual.

Also being questioned, in ways that further corroborate Callon's view of translation, is whether the effects that are being assembled represent *genetic* problems. The neophytes are being exercised in these practices of differentiation and its associated technologies – search engines, databases and photographs of faces and other body parts, histories, chromosome printouts, and so on and so forth.

'Deep play'[1]

Clifford Geertz (1973), the noted cultural anthropologist, talks about the occasions when the ethnographer returns from the field and faces his scientific community in front of 'the blackboard', or rather the whiteboard as it would be called today. The London meeting is the whiteboard of the dysmorphology clinic writ large, the occasion in which members of this growing profession return from the field and perform its special gaze in front of each other.

What is surprising about this academic meeting of the London Dysmorphology Club is the number of cases being presented as interesting but which are then left as unsettled. Their diagnosis appears uncertain. On these, Professor Fox opens the discussion to the audience, asking them to comment and debate, even guess what the diagnosis might be.

At the lunch break I introduce myself to both Professor Smart and to Professor Fox and arrange to contact them for interviews. They are standing talking to someone introduced to me as a scientist. Later on in the London meeting, this scientist presents his research on experiments with mouse mutants.

This is very typical of such meetings – the juxtaposition of the laboratory science and the presentation of the clinical cases. As I have noted earlier 'boundary work' helps keep these matters separate but in ways that give credence to the translation view over the diffusion model.

As I go on to argue later, what is being put on display here is not just clinical certainty but also *uncertainty*. While this meeting is a part of the front of dysmorphology, to enact a medical gaze through which bodies of congenital deformity can be known, the dysmorphologists also perform the association between the laboratory and the clinic as partial and incomplete.

Crucially, in terms of understanding how medicine works as a science, what is being made central is a method of doubt. Certainty is reserved for the clinical moment, the diagnosis of a syndrome. Yet even here, as we have already seen, there is room for doubt. So much so that, like Easter, the clinical moment becomes a moveable feast.

Laboratory technology

The rise of laboratory science in the 19th and 20th centuries appeared to separate itself off from medicine and shift the locus of medical science away from the clinic. Supposedly medical science moved to the laboratory on the one hand and to epidemiology (and statistically based science) on the other. Here the relationship between the clinic and science could be (re)presented in a similar way to the relation between the farm and the laboratory in Latour's study (1988) of the pasteurization of France; that is as 'remote control' (Cooper 1992), with the laboratory establishing itself as a 'centre of calculation' (Latour 1987).

Within this view – contrary to the image we gained through the meeting of the London Dysmorphology Club – the clinic is remote and not involved in the production of medical knowledge. Rather, the pressure is for clinical staff to apply knowledge, determined elsewhere, to efface complexity and heterogeneity (Berg 1992) and to make decisions and 'dispose' of patients (Latimer 1997) at an ever-increasing speed. Thus, the contemporary clinic tends to be reconstituted as a site of intervention in which science is merely consumed within complete clinical episodes. The point is not that grids and codes are abandoned within the clinic. Instead, the rather false idea is that illness and disease are harnessed and sedimented within these classificatory systems, the diagnoses of which are in turn 'carried out' in laboratory tests. There are several problems with this view.

Representing the clinic as remote hides the place of the clinic in the development of laboratory science and technology, and vice versa. Keating and Cambrosio (2003), for example, have demonstrated that historical accounts of the 'new genetics' have been markedly, and inaccurately, skewed: significant advances are attributed to basic sciences and laboratory work, while major contributions arising from clinical research and practice are marginalized or ignored. They suggest that even sociologically sophisticated narratives, like Fujimura's genealogy of oncogene research (Fujimura 1996), imply a linear model of development whereby basic research impacts upon clinical practice (cf. Gaudillière 1993). In contrast, Keating and Cambrosio (2003) conclude rhetorically: 'Could we not say that in many respects clinical research and practice are constitutive of the new genetics and not some kind of passive receptacle awaiting impact?' (p.352).

Keating and Cambrosio extend their reflections to develop their model of 'biomedical platforms', which they understand to be new forms of knowledge not grounded exclusively in either the biological or the clinical. They argue that their model provides a means of capturing the emergence of a new way of making knowledge in the period after World War II that transcends the divide between the normal and the pathological, creating new 'truly biomedical entities' that exist simultaneously as normal biological phenomena and pathological signs. They define biomedical platforms as 'material and discursive arrangements that act as the bench upon which conventions concerning the biological or normal are connected with conventions concerning the medical or pathological' (2003, p.332). This model stresses the intersection of the laboratory, the clinic, industry and mechanisms of regulation in networks of interdependence. The discursive history of medical genetics is a case in point.

The paths of genetic medicine

Medical genetics is a relatively new discipline, probably in the region of 50 years old (Harper 2008), and was only formally recognized as a medical specialty in the US about 30 years ago (Korf 2002). Genetic medicine developed out of human genetics, particularly from the middle of the 20th century.

Its early roots are in understandings from Mendelian genetics, and the identification of pathologies that are inherited, also called single gene disorders. In 1966 Dr Victor A. McKusick, sometimes referred to as the father of medical genetics, wrote his seminal textbook *Mendelian Inheritance in Man; A Catalogue of Human Genes and Genetic Disorders* (1998).[2] In this book McKusick also predicted the mapping of the human genome.

Within this classification system different diseases are listed alongside their gene symbol and their chromosomal location. Some diseases have many clinical differentials so there need to be subcategories. Take Alzheimer's disease as an example: there are 12 different entries for Alzheimer's disease in the OMIM database, some of which share the same chromosomal location and gene labels, and others which do not.

Currently there are very interesting developments in this process through which clinical categories, such as Alzheimer's disease, appear to be being refigured by new understandings of the chromosomal and genetic relation between what were originally considered 'separate' diagnoses, prompting the possibility of a revision of clinical classification. An example of this is the spectrum of mental health disorders from autism, schizophrenia, bipolar disorders through to Alzheimer's disease, which seem to share some elements at the genetic level.

I want to emphasize an important feature of the kind of clinical work that we are dealing with here: pathological effects described clinically are, in medical genetics, being mapped to genes and their location on chromosomes. Knowledge production, and the relation between science and medicine, is performed in medical genetics very much in terms of a *medical* platform. A part of this process includes refiguring clinical classification of mental and physical disorders, including the parameters of disorders and their etiologies.

This said, the history of the emergence of medical genetics also includes older roots –not in the classification of disease diagnoses, but in the association of human developmental science, and the identification of causes of congenital anomalies, often described as syndromes. As we saw in the Introduction these may include susceptibility to disease, but they are not equivalent to disease.

A science of growth and form

Most of the dysmorphologists I talked to had 'come from' paediatrics, and 'got into genetics' through that route. This disciplinary genealogy is evident in their inclusion of a pregnancy history and a history of the child's development in their presentation of cases at conferences or in papers.

Dysmorphologists also make a distinction between themselves and other kinds of medical geneticists, who have come through the route of disease-orientated genetics, such as cancer genetics. This latter kind of genetics is much more prone to look for the genes that are implicated in the production of the underlying conditions for the disease process, such as Alzheimer's (as discussed above) in which many related genes have been discovered. In contrast, paediatric genetics is much more focussed on the relationship between growth, shape and form and the development of the human organism. The interest in diseases is where these are associated with malformation.

Genetic medicine in dysmorphology is thus not simply concerned with diseases. Rather it has a direct relationship to what I want to delineate as the *science of growth and form*, after D'Arcy Wentworth Thompson (2000). These sciences include morphogenesis, embryology, and developmental biology, on the one hand, and psycho-physiological theories of normal child development on the other. In the natural history of genetic medicine concerned with congenital abnormalities, there is therefore an association between clinical paediatrics and biological theories of human growth and development, including more recently genetics.

There is a long history of people seeking explanations for specific kinds of differences in babies and children (Crawford 2004). In contemporary Euro-American societies, deformity in babies and children has become increasingly medicalized, so that we are used to thinking of differences in terms of 'congenital abnormalities' or 'anomalies', or 'birth defects'. Medicalization has included twin processes: distinguishing when defects have serious, even life-threatening implications, and clinical processes through which effects are identified and named *as* deformities, including creating ways of dividing the normal from the abnormal, and identifying the causes of deformity.

Increasingly, surveillance of children's failure to grow and thrive has been standardized: for example, in tecnologies for measuring and charting growth and form in foetuses, babies and infants, and plotting these results in relation to ranges and norms. There are a number of technologies that can help identify abnormalities in growth and form prenatally – for example, foetal growth percentile calculators – as well as detecting potential abnormalities in the form of the foetus.[3] These technologies can help detect variations. For example, specificities over how a baby fails to grow properly in the womb, are related to how the baby is born with defects such as harelip and cleft palate, too many or not enough fingers or toes, too big or too small a head. Other 'common' failures may include growing too large or being too small for foetal chronological age.

Additionally, deviations from the norm may involve organs – brains may fail to grow in the right way or hearts fail to close up where they should. Birth defects do not always show immediately: they can make their appearance over time as the child is seen to fail to develop 'normally'. Here defects can present over time, such as 'abnormal' behaviour, including what is now categorized as mental retardation, autism and attention deficit hyperactivity disorder.

Medical explanations for birth defects include environmental factors during pregnancy – such as foetal exposure to chemicals, infections (such as rubella), and radiation – or parental lifestyle factors, such as drug consumption (such as alcohol or lithium), as well as events during birth itself, such as lack of oxygen. Some birth defects are identified as having a chromosomal or genetic origin. This can be inherited, from one or both parents, or seen as a de novo event, where there has been an aberration at the chromosomal or genetic level but that this has not been inherited from either parent, although there may be other correlations, for example between Down syndrome and older mothers. Doctors in dysmorphology set out not just to identify the effects of defects, but to differentiate their causes. This is why they do a careful pregnancy and birth history – to exclude any environmental or lifestyle factors that might have affected the child during its development in the womb or during birth, or even after birth.

The geneticization of congenital disorders

Dysmorphology thus has its roots and routes in the description and explanation of deformities, and, as such, has been at the heart of the emergence of medical genetics as a specialism in the UK. In the US, dysmorphology is a distinctive department set apart from medical genetics, while in the UK dysmorphology is located within medical genetics as an integral part of medical and clinical genetics, and as a key underpinning knowledge practice to the discipline.

Specifically, the histories of medical genetics in the UK associate it with, on the one hand, correlating complex human traits and pathologies with hereditary mechanisms (Kaplan 2000), and on the other, with landmark innovative technologies (Harper 2004, 2006), for example chromosome karyotyping.[4]

It has been suggested that the history of medical genetics was in part curtailed because the Eugenics movement associated hereditary and the social – human genetics was promoted as a way to breed people in order to strengthen the race and eliminate 'the weak' (Richards 2002). Dunn (1962) argues that it is only later, when human genetics was rearticulated as of medical importance and as a way to understand 'genetical' problems in individuals as new kinds of medical entities, including the part genetics plays in normal human development and the production of health and pathology, that a renaissance and flourishing of human genetic science was possible:

> Progress in human genetics seemed to have been impeded less by lack of means than by lack of a clear scientific goal, and this at a time when the major problems of genetics were taking a clear form. *The particulate nature of the transmission mechanism of heredity had focused attention on the means by which genetic elements reproduce and maintain their continuity with opportunity for change and evolution, and on the means by which genes control metabolism and development. But most observations on human heredity were not oriented in any clear way toward such problems.* Matters of greater moment seemed to be the inheritance of 'insanity,' of 'feeblemindedness' and other then vaguely defined mental ills, the effects of parental age or alcoholism or social status on the offspring, and similar studies pursued for immediate social ends.
>
> (p.2, emphasis added)

Critically, then, the emergence of the technologies with which to visualize chromosomal, and later gene, sequences, have helped legitimate the differentiation of genetic as opposed to other kinds of aetiologies, for variation and difference in growth and form associated with complex human troubles. As I have discussed in Chapter 3, medicalization of human variation as deformity has helped legitimate the need for the technoscience.

Thus the study of complex human troubles, defined as congenital, already has a long history, together with a history of differentiating their origins, including environment, perinatal events, such as alcohol consumption during pregnancy, and so on and so forth. Here I should stress two things. The first is how the medical history of complex human troubles identified as congenital, and their association with heredity, reproduction and family, has legitimated the development of the technologies with which to visualize them. The second is that the development of technologies to 'visualize' the chromosomes and the genes has legitimated the rapid and proliferating interest in the description of congenital abnormalities – or 'syndromes'. This relation between medicine and science is increasingly sedimented in Euro-American health policy.

To elaborate: recently the American College of Medical Genetics (Watson *et al.* 2006), in a policy directive, advocated screening at birth for 29 different conditions, including many syndromes with a 'genetic' origin. Further sedimentation can be found in registers for congenital anomalies. Across regions and nations in Europe, as well as states in the US, information about congenital anomalies is collected on a vast scale to form a database for statistical analysis of deformity at the level of populations. In Europe these registers are gathered together by EUROCAT (http://www.eurocat-network.eu/aboutus/whatiseurocat/whyregistercongenitalanomalies). These reporting mechanisms include reporting of anomalies that have chromosomal and genetic causes.

Hidden in all this is how any specific syndrome has emerged; how it comes to be classified and defined, and continuously refined, prior to its naturalization in a test, or a policy, or as a diagnosis and reportable event. For example, the work of classifying chromosomal anomalies, such as Down syndrome or Turner syndrome, has been sedimented and naturalized in the technologies with which to visualize them at the molecular level.

This process can be seen in antenatal and newborn screening programmes. For some time both in the UK, Europe and the US pregnant mothers are routinely offered screening for Down syndrome. Down syndrome has been medicalized through the association of visible features with problems of growth and development, as well as with some diseases:

> Though the symptoms of Down syndrome are very dangerous, it is possible that the patients won't experience all of them. Most of them are morphological abnormalities like asymmetrical, small skull, abnormal round head with a flat side at the back. Besides, a child with Down syndrome can have slanting eyes, short hands (sometimes broad) and fingers. The nose is usually flattened, the mouth is small with an enlarged tongue (which causes serious problems). The children with Down syndrome also have low muscle tone (which cause feeding problems) and loose joints. Besides the rate of weight increase at the DS newborns is slower than the normal newborns. Unfortunately DS affects also the mental abilities of the child. DS patients suffer from moderate mental retardation. Besides, these newborns face problems in developing some skills like feeding, toilet teaching etc. Besides there is a positive connection between Down syndrome and Alzheimer and Leukaemia.
>
> (Genetic Diseases, undated)

Down syndrome is now also sometimes called trisomy 21. This is because its diagnosis was 'settled' in 1959 by tests that have allowed it to be seen as a chromosomal condition caused by the presence of all or part of an extra 21st chromosome. As it happens, Down syndrome was originally named after a British physician who described the syndrome in 1866. What is interesting is that in the US the syndrome is now actually called trisomy 21 – this technoscientific labelling thus effacing the trace of its clinical origins as something 'discovered' by Dr Down. Indeed, the shift from an eponymous (Brighton and Brighton 1987) naming of syndromes to a name that designates the gene or the chromosome is becoming more prevalent. This is itself significant in greatly masking the *clinical* part played in the development of genetic technology.

I should add here that Down syndrome is one of the original dysmorphic syndromes with its own special 'look', both in terms of facial features and the shape and form of hands and feet (see Figure 4.3).

In this brief history we can see the intertwining and co-dependency of clinical knowledge creation and genetic science in the context of understandings about congenital abnormalities. Because congenital abnormality is being figured as a problem of growth and form, clinical work is deeply entangled in shifts in biosciences and vice a versa, including the development of biotechnologies such as karyotyping. These relations and associations, or 'assemblages' (Collier and Ong 2005), become invisible once they are stabilized as diagnostic categories and sedimented as screening technologies, such as those for Down and Turner syndromes.

Critically, recognized expert dysmorphologists are the key actors in the construction and dissemination of databases of abnormalities – and the construction of clinical entities that may or may not be screenable in the future. Some of these experts form the subjects of the current study. But what is being performed in dysmorphology is the messiness of categorical work (Bowker and Star 2000) in the making. And, as will be seen, it is in this messiness that dysmorphology enacts clinical observation and classification of Sean B. Carroll's 'spectacular

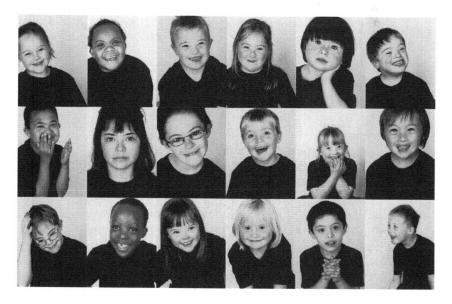

Figure 4.3 The many faces of Down syndrome: Richard Bailey *365* (2008). Reproduced with kind permission of Richard Bailey.

mutants' that occur 'in nature' as opposed to in the laboratory, as necessary to the science of the new genetics.

Genetics and (de)formation: from correlations to causes

Within the medical genetics concerned with anomalies in growth and form, a child's development is explored at the molar level of the whole organism: namely, at the clinical level. With changes in biological understanding, it follows that there are changes in clinical possibilities: that is, with a proliferation of genetic science and technology, the question of whether the clinical picture is a phenotype (the fleshy expression of a genotype) is increasingly opened up. This is referred to as the phenotype-genotype correlation:

> The distinction between phenotype and genotype is fundamental to the understanding of heredity and development of organisms. The *genotype* of an organism is the class to which that organism belongs as determined by the description of the actual physical material made up of DNA that was passed to the organism by its parents at the organism's conception. For sexually reproducing organisms [such as humans] that physical material consists of the DNA contributed to the fertilized egg by the sperm and egg of its two parents. The *phenotype* of an organism is the class to which that organism belongs as determined by the description of the physical and behavioral characteristics of the organism, for example its size and shape, its metabolic activities and its pattern of movement. It is essential to distinguish the descriptors of the organism, its genotype and phenotype, from the material objects that are being described. The genotype is the descriptor of the *genome*, which is the set of physical DNA molecules inherited from the organism's parents. The phenotype is the descriptor of the *phenome*, the manifest physical properties of the organism, its physiology, morphology and behavior. The concepts of phenotype and genotype also demand the distinction between *types* and *tokens*. As the words 'genotype' and 'phenotype' suggest, these are types, sets of which any given organism and its genome are members, sets defined by their physical description. *Any individual organism and its genome are members of those sets, tokens of those types.*
>
> (*Stanford Encyclopedia of Philosophy* 2004, emphasis added)

It is interesting to note that features of a phenotype do not necessarily correlate to a genotype: these features can express different genotypes. As can be seen from the above quotation, the individual organism and its genome can become members of a 'class' or 'set', or be held up as representing a 'token of a type'. Here, then, we are not talking about direct causal relations, or the discovery of truth or laws, but about *correlations*, based on associations that have to be evidenced rather than proven:

> The association between the presence of a certain mutation or mutations (genotype) and the resulting physical trait, abnormality, or pattern of

abnormalities (phenotype). With respect to genetic testing, the frequency with which a certain phenotype is observed in the presence of a specific genotype determines the positive predictive value of the test.

(U.S. National Library of Medicine, National Institutes of Health)

The predictive value of any particular molecular test is gained not in demonstrating causal relations, but through correlations between what is observed (phenotype) and the presence of a particular genotype – in other words there has to be observation of a phenotype ahead of a) its sedimentation in a classification system and b) its correlation with a specific genotype represented by a test. Therefore, the advent of the new genetics opens up a new site: the relation and non-relation between the molecular (the genotype) and the molar (the phenotype).

This relationship between the observation, description and validation of a phenotype, and its correlation to a specific genotype, is the space occupied by the dysmorphology clinic in genetic medicine. The relationship between clinical genetic medicine and the science of human growth and development is of some standing, and its incorporation of new genetic knowledge in terms of both the classification of congenital abnormalities (as well as in the recognition, diagnosis and 'treatment' of congenital abnormalities) is ongoing. In the main, this can be understood as a process through which there has to be an arrival at a position in which *correlations can be tested* in the establishing of genetic etiologies.

Classification in dysmorphology

A key site in which this work is being undertaken is dysmorphology, and the formation of a particular kind of discourse and particular kind of gaze. In the ways that dysmorphology classification is presented, knowledge about the origins of a syndrome comes after its original description.

In terms of the medical model, this represents the reductive process of medical categorizing: the move is from correlations to causes. This includes a shift from the clinical observation and description of syndromes to the laboratory and the experimental mode through which to discover the underlying defects causing the syndrome:

> The biochemical and physiological defects underlying human dysmorphic syndromes can now be approached using techniques of molecular biology. The genetic component of the causation of the dysmorphology can be studied in isolation from the environmental component by using large, rare families that exhibit the same phenotype as more complex multifactorial disorders, but inherit the mutation in a monogenic fashion. Such an analysis starts with the determination of linkage to a gene probe, followed by the use of *newer techniques of molecular biology to enable cloning and sequencing of the mutated gene.* Analysis of the gene product by amino acid sequence homology to other known proteins, and tissue specific expression, may place the defect within the cascade of events associated with development and differentiation.

Once cloned, the gene can also be manipulated in transgenic laboratory animals and the effect of its mutation studied directly. The use of techniques of molecular biology to study the genetic aspects of dysmorphic syndromes will allow insight to be gained both into normal foetal development and into the causes of congenital malformations.

(Ivens *et al.* 1988, p.473, emphasis added)

As already indicated, most of the experts I encountered in the study were also involved in collaborative research with laboratory-based scientists trying to identify the genetic basis of syndromes. These laboratories (both cytogenic and molecular genetic laboratories) were situated alongside the clinics. They provided not just clinical investigative services, but also acted as homes for collaborative work between clinical and laboratory-based scientists. For example, one medical genetics department and its associated molecular genetics laboratory had been intimately involved together in cloning the myotonic dystrophy and Huntington gene for which diagnostic tests and family follow up is now routine. In addition, at many of the meetings I attended, laboratory-based research using animal models or clones would be presented alongside the presentation of dysmorphology case studies. In the lobby of national and international human or medical genetics conferences, posters would be mixed together displaying clinical case studies and laboratory research, sometimes the two being juxtaposed within the same poster.

What is being enacted here then is how contemporary discovery in clinically orientated genetic science contravenes any notion that new genetic knowledge follows a diffusion model – from bench to bedside – but relies rather on the intermingling of clinical and laboratory work in the co-constitution of genetic knowledge. Indeed, as I have suggested, classification of syndromes as genetic, or not, is performed in dysmorphology as very much still in the making (Latimer *et al.* 2006). This is corroborated by Featherstone and Atkinson (2011) who also show, in their recent study of Rhett syndrome as a syndrome in the making, activities in one domain (the clinic) influence perception in the other (the laboratory).

This refutes the usual way in which the flow of innovation is represented. Indeed, even where there are conscious attempts at correlating descriptions of a phenotype (in the clinic) and visualization of the corresponding genotype (in the laboratory), there can be a gap between the two. This gap in the correlation between phenotype and genotype is a feature of how genetics and the classification of syndromes proceeds, one that is captured by Morris (2006) in the opening of her chapter on the dysmorphology, natural history and genetics of Williams syndrome (see Figure 4.4).

She suggests that 'The study of a syndrome typically proceeds in a stepwise fashion reflecting distinct knowledge increments', including a linear and progressive process from clinical discovery of a unique pattern through to definition of a condition, cataloguing of the natural history, delineation of the causes of the syndrome, including teratogens, mutant genes and chromosome abnormalities, and finally genotype-phenotype correlation. This latter phase, or 'knowledge increment', is described by Morris as when:

- The population of clinically affected individuals is examined. With an objective test for diagnosis, researchers can detect both extremes (mild and severe) of the distribution, resulting in a redefinition of the syndrome.
- The range of the phenotype is better evaluated.
- Researchers investigate the variability in phenotype relative to the particular genetic mutation, the genetic background, varying environmental conditions and the actions of modifying genes.
- Genetic heterogeneity may be demonstrated for the phenotype, if a mutation in a different gene is found to result in the same clinical syndrome.

(Morris 2006, p.3)

Morris is asserting that the laboratory work can help refine the clinical description of a syndrome, including reevaluating the range (mild to severe), and even help redefine classification where different mutations result in the same clinical picture. This is very much a picture of translation rather than diffusion in the relation between the laboratory and the clinic in the description and refining

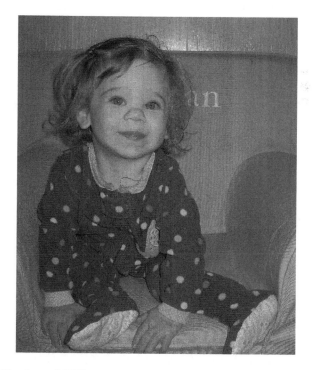

Figure 4.4 The face of Williams syndrome. Reproduced with kind permission of The Williams Syndrome Association, http://www.williams-syndrome.org/

of syndromes. Critically, however, it also indicates a gap – what I want to call a possible non-relation between the visualization of the genotype and the clinical picture of a phenotype. Also missing from this account is how, for many clinical descriptions, there is as yet no way of visualizaing the genotype. I return to describe how clinicians account for this process in Chapter 5.

Discussion

In this chapter I have shown that what is being performed by the association of the clinic with the laboratory, as well as with technoscientific representations of genes and chromosomes, is the possibility of new knowledge and understanding about disease. We have seen, in discourses about the history of medical genetics and the natural histories of syndromes, the figuring of what Keating and Cambrosio (2003) describe as *medical platforms* in the creation of new medical entities.

This is important because the recurrent motif in the expanding research literature on the relation between science and medicine – in the context of the so-called geneticization of contemporary medicine – is a scepticism concerning reductionist explanations of medical knowledge (cf. Kerr 2004a, pp.24–8). It has been stressed that there is a need to avoid the assumption that medical knowledge and practice can be accounted for either in terms of increasing molecularization (e.g. de Chadarevian and Kamminga 1998), or in the rise of technology (e.g. Wailoo 1997).

Kerr's (2000) exploration of cystic fibrosis is a key case in point. She demonstrates the flexibility of genes and disease entities in the complex intersections between genetic and clinical research. While genetic reductionism is a feature of much of the scientific and medical texts she examines, she argues for social-science analyses that 'contextualize genetic reductionism' (p.870), stressing the 'variability and contingency' that characterize the accomplishment of genetic categorizations.

The consequent dialogue between Kerr and Hedgecoe (Hedgecoe 2003, 2004a; Kerr 2004b) serves to underscore the fact that, while social scientists may wish to treat 'geneticization' as a topic for inquiry (as reflected in the rhetoric and practices of scientists and clinicians), it should not be invoked as an unexamined explanation for current practice (see Hedgecoe 2002; Hedgecoe and Tutton 2002; Gibbon 2002). Cox and Starzomski (2004), discussing the construction of autosomal dominant polycystic kidney disease, also argue that the complexities of everyday practice escape simple characterizations as 'geneticization'. There are, of course, wider cultural analyses in which the notion of geneticization has been invoked to account for generic consequences of the new genetics (e.g. Finkler 2000) and to contest strong versions of a geneticized 'medicalization' thesis (Cussins 1996; Lock and Kaufert 1998; Martin 1998).

Conclusion

In this chapter I have examined the various discourses over dysmorphology's contribution to genetic science. These fit neatly with Foucault's analysis of medicine as an enlightenment project and the emphasis on the naturalist's gaze, discussed in Chapter 2, in which 'observation should lead to experiment, provided that experiment should question only in the vocabulary and within the language proposed to it by things observed' (Foucault 2003a, p.131).

However, I am suggesting that there is a greater significance here. This extra significance concerns, first, the gap between the phenotype and the genotype as well as the partialness of the relationality between the molar and the molecular. And, second, it concerns how dysmorphology performs the relation between the normal and the pathological in understandings of human growth and development as *emergent*.

In the next chapter I go on to suggest how these (partial) relations are accomplished in dysmorphology. My argument is that these pressage the clinic in genetics as a new frontier of knowledge – site in which medicine, albeit incipiently, might be thought to be beginning to reassert its dominance in society.

5 Shaping the science of growth and form

The constant division between the normal and the abnormal, to which every individual is subjected, brings us back to our own time, by applying the binary branding and exile of the leper to quite different objects; the existence of a whole set of techniques and institutions for measuring, supervising and correcting the abnormal brings into play the disciplinary mechanisms to which the fear of the plague gave rise. All the mechanisms of power which, even today, are disposed around the abnormal individual, to brand him and to alter him, are composed of those two forms [the plague and the leper] from which they distantly derive.

(Foucault 1995, p.199)

Introduction

In the last chapter I began to examine how clinical geneticists lay claim to the science of growth and form, exploring how the genealogy of dysmorphology is also a history of the medicalization of deformity in children, one that is critical to the emergence of genetic medicine in the late 20th and early 21st centuries. This included looking at how developments in molecular biology intertwine with clinical medicine's history and interest in how the genetic is implicated in the production of congenital abnormalities, or syndromes.

In this chapter I explore further how the clinical identification and description of pathologies takes place. My aim is to begin to explore in detail how the shape of forms for congenitally *abnormal* entities connects to how the genetic is being investigated as playing a part in *normal* human development. It is this work of dividing the normal from the abnormal that is, as Foucault suggests in the citation above, an underpinning mechanism of power, a mechanism through which the clinic reinforces its authority.

Donnai (2008), a leading British dysmorphologist, states in a lecture to neophyte geneticists that: 'David Smith from the USA first used the term "dysmorphology" in the 1960s to describe the study of human congenital malformations and patterns of birth defects'. She goes on to add that dysmorphology is important for both families and for our understanding of human development. In this statement she is making the claim that by studying the abnormal and the pathological, we can understand much more about the normal. Or to put it another way: by studying 'morphological defects' we can learn more about normal human development.

In the following, I elaborate how this process of relating the abnormal to the normal may be working through an analysis of an extract from my interview with Professor Smart. Ahead of this, however, I note some similarities and differences between the academic meetings of dysmorphology and earlier displays of medical dominance, particularly in terms of its warrant to identify and divide the normal and the abnormal.

Staging the display

Occasions such as the London Dysmorphology Club described in the previous chapter conjure up visions of 'grand rounds', the ritual events in which medical case histories were presented as a vital part of medical education and science. Grand rounds took place in auditoriums located either in the teaching hospital or in the medical school – often designed for that purpose, with steep sides and a circular central floor. Usually the patient that formed the focus of the case was present, and their history and treatment presented, and then debated by members of the audience at great length.

The grand round constituted the 'deep play' (Geertz 1973) at the heart of clinical medicine and was where medicine was visualized and reaffirmed *as* grand. In the grand round what was at stake was much more than the enactment of an empirically grounded discipline of discovery and innovation. What was being put on display was a competitive and hierarchical world in which doctors more or less produced and reproduced medical perception, judgement and discretion.

Grand rounds, like the ones I used to attend at University College and St Mary's Hospitals in London, were just such sites for the spectacle of medical dominance to be re-enacted. Teaching ward rounds at the bedside were also such occasions although not on such a large scale. However, they could still be spectacles of the medical gaze, hierarchy and competition, and the method of doubt, with sometimes up to 30 attendants, including visiting doctors from all over the world. Increasingly, however, with audit cultures, political correctness and technologies of democratization (such as pathways, evidence-based medicine and patient choice) it would appear that medicine is in retreat, becoming almost recessive, with only intermittent displays of dominance (cf. Latimer 2004). For example, a doctor in the *New York Times* (Altman 2006) suggested that while some leading medical schools now stream and podcast what they call grand rounds for public consumption (e.g. the Mayo clinic @ http://www.mayoclinic.org/grand-rounds/), grand rounds as a space for Socratic dialogue has been lost.

In conjuring up these contrasting images, I want to press three things. The first is how the meeting of the London Dysmorphology Club is one of medicine's 'fronts' (Goffman 1980). Its mimicry of the grand round of old offers an occasion in which dysmorphology is magnified, enacted, circulated and passed on.

The fact that the spectacle of medical dominance is displayed only intermittently today makes such theatre no less potent. Secondly, the presenters are often neophytes rather than established clinicians. The career young are being exercised and disciplined through their participation, not merely through witnessing as members of the audience.

Thirdly, and perhaps most importantly, the meeting also acts as an occasion that contemporizes the power of the medical gaze through the specificities of its technologies and practices. However, in place of the fleshy bodies that constituted the focus of the grand round, it is assemblages and syndromes displayed on twin screens that magnify the modus operandi of dysmorphology. In this virtual world, the patient is made present only occasionally and remotely through visual recognition and oral histories.

Genetic medicine and the science of growth and form

As reported in my description of the London Dysmorphology Club in Chapter 4, Professor Smart is the man who was sitting at his laptop, sending images and database to the screen on the left of the podium. Later he tells me a story that elaborates how medicine brings the clinic, the laboratory and the family into association. Critically, Professor Smart's story emphasizes the clinic's place in generating knowledge about growth and form in humans, in a way that captures how he, and other experts I interviewed, present the relation between the clinic and the laboratory in processes of discovery and innovation.

The interview is taking place in the café of the same building in which the London Dysmorphology Club was held. As it happens I never get behind this front to the backstage of his office – or gain access to his clinic or laboratories (also housed in this building) – possibly because with his laptop he brings much of his backstage with him wherever he goes.

As he talks to me, Professor Smart is showing me pictures and articles and all sorts of data on his laptop. During the whole interview, the mouse of his computer is competing for space with the coffee cups and my tape recorder on the café table. This has a certain irony since one of my questions leads to the topic of laboratory mice coming to dominate his narrative on the natural history of Fraser syndrome:

JL: Just one more technical thing before you take me through the [dysmorphology] database, which is mouse modelling, and how does that help clinical work or, what's your view if you like?

PROFESSOR SMART: Mice don't really have much clinically, but they do help in research, to give clues as to where a gene might be. One of the things that we've done very recently, on the research side, is a good example of how useful mice are. I've always been interested in mice, so I've actually got a database that is equivalent to the human database, which is a database of mouse mutants, of abnormal mice. I'll show you that in a minute. Let's show you how mice are useful. This is a slightly gory picture, okay – this is a syndrome called Fraser's syndrome. [He shows me some slides, pictures of a blind mouse as well as pictures of children with blinded eyes – see Figure 5.1.]

(Author interview, 2003–2004)

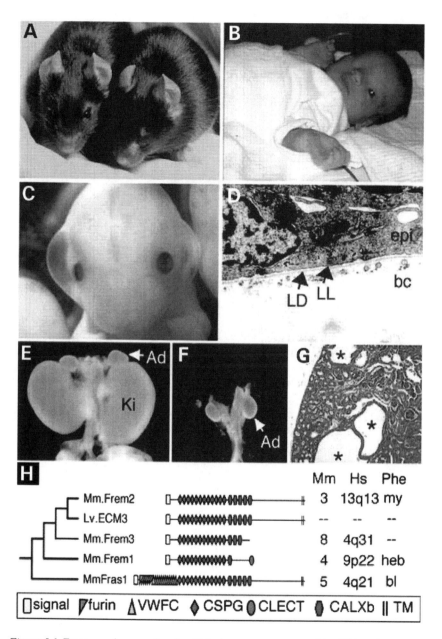

Figure 5.1 Fraser syndrome – showing blebs in mouse mutants and in children (Smyth and Scambler 2005). Reproduced with kind permission of the Oxford University Press.

Professor Smart begins this part of the interview with a distinction between the fact that mice don't have much to offer clinically and the significance of their place in genetic research, in that they are good at helping you find the genes. In Latour's terms (1987) Professor Smart is mobilizing mice as 'spokespersons' not for clinical anomalies, but for their genetic basis. So here we have the doubling that the clinic performs: as a site of knowledge production about the genes and their functions, and as a site in which diseases are classified, diagnosed and intervened in.

Professor Smart goes on to say that he has a database of mouse mutants and their abnormalities, and that he can show me how mice are useful. He then shows me some pictures of the blinded eyes of mice and human mutants – note the overlap and the distinction between mice and humans. As he continues, he shifts between his talk and the different images on his laptop:

PROFESSOR SMART: It is named after a guy called George Fraser, who was an *old-time geneticist*, in Oxford. Fraser syndrome – slightly gory – [returns to the slides of the images of mice and people with Fraser syndrome] – the eyelids don't actually form, so cryptothalamus – hidden eyes – so they don't actually have any eye openings, and underneath there, even if you open them up surgically, the eyeball is not normal, so they are blind basically. And the other thing they have is ... syndactyly – their fingers are joined together. Here is George's original paper [he brings up a pdf of the original paper on his screen], so this is *way back in 1962*.

(Emphasis added)

Here Professor Smart is implicitly making another distinction – George Fraser was an 'old-time geneticist'; as if to corroborate this designation, he shows me the original paper that was published 'way back' in 1962. He enacts Fraser syndrome as being discovered through observation of nature, in 'the field' of the family, and identification of clinical signs and unusual features, which the special clinical gaze associates with one another (eyes, joined-up fingers) published in an early paper by Dr Fraser.

In doing this Professor Smart begins to historicize, and give a sense of discovery and progress – a sense that he is describing the 'natural' history of an evolving clinical medicine, but one that is also engaged in discovery over the genetic. He then goes on to tell me a 'funny story':

PROFESSOR SMART: This is a funny story – this lady here [shows me a slide of a woman in her forties], she's got cryptothalamus and she is obviously aged about 45, and her mum, who was aged about 70 wrote to me, just out of the blue because she didn't know I was working on Fraser syndrome. And she said 'I've always wondered what was wrong with my daughter and somebody has said that she's got Charge syndrome'.[1] So I said, 'Well I don't know, but send us some pictures'. So she sent some – and I said 'Oh well

I think we do know what she's got, perhaps you'd like to come to the clinic and we can talk to you'. Talked to her and said it was something called Fraser syndrome, and she said 'Oh that's funny because somebody called Dr Fraser came to see us about 40 years ago!' And it turns out this is the original case from the paper [by Dr Fraser], although nobody had told her what he was going to do, but anyway.

JL: So did he not go back to them?

PROFESSOR SMART: I don't know. But she didn't know that this was Fraser syndrome and this was the original case. So anyway it is recessive, and it is quite difficult, this lady has obviously survived, but a lot of them die early on because they get absent kidneys and they get blocked larynxes – so... it is quite difficult to get cases, DNA, genetic studies, so there aren't many cases around.

Professor Smart in this section goes on to describe how, through serendipity, he gets to re-examine the original case of Fraser syndrome. He enacts the 'gestalt', or instant recognition, of the gaze in dysmorphology – he had asked the mother to send some pictures and then he knew what she and the daughter had. But then he expresses something different – how the mother and her daughter become interesting to him because the mother had survived, while in fact the syndrome is quite difficult – people often die early. He mentions the genetics – it is recessive – but because of these early deaths doing genetic studies on the DNA of affected families is problematic.

Yet, as Professor Smart goes on to illuminate, the point of his story is not the curiosity of his meeting the mother, or of her mere survival:

PROFESSOR SMART: I was hanging on for about 15 years, because there's a group of mice called the Bleb mutant mice, which look like Fraser syndrome [shows me a slide of a mouse] – and you can't see – but they haven't got open eyelids either, and they've got syndactyly, and they are called Bleb mutant mice [see Figure 5.1] because – this is a mouse embryo – early on in development, they get these blebs or blisters and these are like sort of blood blisters really, and you see that one sitting over the eyeball, and that one sitting over the lower limb part, so it is thought that they interfere mechanically with the development of the eyeball.

JL: And that's a naturally occurring mouse – so to speak?

PROFESSOR SMART: It is –

JL: As opposed to an engineered one?

PROFESSOR SMART: Yes, that's one [slide of a mouse with bleb eyes] that has been collected a long time ago because it looked interesting. In fact – this is … I got taught about mice in the 1960s by a guy called Grüneberg,[2] who was a middle-European man, who spent his whole life looking at mice, and he thought it was pretty weird, and I should have listened to him a little harder. So this is from his book from about the 1950s [shows me a slide of a cross section of a mouse's eyeball], showing a cross section of an eyeball and these mice with their blebs – that's the eyelid that didn't form, and that's the blister and that's the eyeball. So they've known about them for a long time. But the thing is that in the mouse there are different genes that cause the same picture, so there are at least five genes, which means it's heterogeneous, and that tells us it is going to be very difficult to map it in the humans, because you get a load of families, but you are not just looking at the one locus, the one gene, you might be looking at four genes, which means in terms of genetic mapping it makes it extremely difficult, if not impossible. But if you've got these clues from the mouse, it helps. So the thing is these mice have been [useful]. *If we breed the mice, they can all be mapped pretty easily to specific mouse chromosomes, so we didn't know what the gene was in the mouse but we knew what chromosome it was on.*

(Emphasis added)

In this passage he invokes the length of time it took to move the genetics of Fraser syndrome along: 'I was hanging on for about 15 years'. And here he switches from the family with Fraser syndrome to his attachment to mice, and the history of another discovery: a particular kind of mouse that also has eye problems identical to people with Fraser syndrome.

In the same passage, he then proceeds to give a history of how mapping the genes in the mice gave clues. He is implying that while it is hard to do gene mapping studies in humans, if mice are bred (with the mutation) they can be mapped pretty easily – not to the genes – since 'there are at least five genes' – but to the chromosomes.

The significance of this point begins to emerge when Professor Smart goes on with his natural history of discovering the genetics of Fraser syndrome:

And what we can do is … here we are [shows me a slide] – this is something called the Oxford grid. It turns out that although mice have got 20 chromosomes, 20 pairs of chromosomes and humans have got 23, and they look different down the microscope, chunks of mouse chromosome are conserved – so if you look at the genes on one particular mouse chromosome it will all be in the same chunk in the humans. So in this recent paper here – so that is the human chromosome – 7 – and there is a.. mouse [chromosome] … so for example this bit of human 7, all the genes there are the same as the ones on the bit of mouse 5 – and a little bit of mouse 6. So it means that if – let's say a gene has been mapped with a bit of mouse 6 syndrome, it is a good first guess that it might be on this bit of chromosome 7 – but if you don't know that, you have to do what is called a [...] gene-linkage approach, which is when you have to use markers – 300 markers for every chromosome and if you haven't got very many families then you probably can't do that. So it is useful to have a clue like this [the mouse mutants]. So because we knew which mouse chromosomes these genes were on, then we could have a guess as to where the human's were.

In this passage of his story Professor Smart explains the relation between how the laboratory mapping of chromosomes in mice works to give clues as to where to look in humans. Here we enter the world of the molecular. We are in a new landscape to that of blebs, joined-up fingers and problem kidneys. We are in a landscape of chromosomes, genome sequencing and genetic maps, one that is able to compare mice and humans. What happens on chromosome 5 and 6 in the mouse, because of the technology known as the Oxford grid,[3] a technology that compares maps of human genomes with those of mice, Professor Smart can suggest that Fraser syndrome might be something that happens on chromosome 7 in humans. Of course chromosome 7 in humans is made up of hundreds of genes. But, as he puts it, it gives us a clue.

As he continues, he switches extensions in his discourse – back from mice, and the Oxford grid, to families, and on to 'knock-out' or genetically engineered mice:

PROFESSOR SMART: Then we got some inbred families which are also useful for mapping and got those – a Pakistani family up in Leeds and Bradford – they are very helpful for those mapping studies, because they – if they do have a problem like this [Fraser syndrome] then you can have it affecting multiple members in the family. So then we mapped it and we found the gene basically. This is a mouse – now this is a knockout mouse[4] – somebody else knocked out this mouse and produced exactly the same picture with these blebs. So that was useful with the mice because it told us that there was more than one locus involved and it helped us to find the gene because we knew which bit of the chromosome to look at. Now of course, we've got a mouse model to try and understand what else is going on. Because it is a rather novel protein, so it is one of those things, where nobody had found that protein before in humans – it hadn't been found because of Fraser syndrome – but obviously when it is working normally it was doing something important in the mouse skin as well. It is also odd because these mice and humans have absent kidneys as well sometimes, and that is not caused by the … *so it [the gene/protein] is doing something important in kidney development* [emphasis added].

JL: So something else is going on.

PROFESSOR SMART: So yes, mice have helped there.

JL: That's really useful.

PROFESSOR SMART: I've got a project too – as I say we've got this mouse database but we want to link up our database of the mouse with this [our human database], so that we can get clues more efficiently basically.

JL: So it sort of helps you to know where to look – that's partly how?

PROFESSOR SMART: And then it helps you to find the mouse model for one human disease.

In this final passage of his story, Professor Smart tells me about how they then 'got some inbred Pakistani families' and mapped their genes and discovered the gene for Fraser syndrome. But then he switches his focus on human bodies back to the mice – it was the 'mouse model', the knock-out mouse engineered to 'model' Fraser syndrome, which helped them locate the gene: it helped them know that there was more 'than one locus'.

The experimental laboratory-based science in the form of the engineered mouse, which becomes a 'mouse model', is thus helping in more than the clinical understanding of Fraser syndrome. The natural history of Fraser syndrome, the switching between people – the mother and her daughter, the Pakistani families – the mice (the original mutant mice), and then the transgenic knock-out mice that someone else made that had the same blebs – is, in Professor Smart's account, critically not just key to discovering the genetics of a syndrome. Rather, in moving from the family to the transgenic mouse, he suggests that they have created a mouse model of Fraser syndrome, with the specific genes on chromosome 7 and, therefore, making not just gene mapping, but experimental work possible. This is articulated as important, not simply in terms of one human developmental disease, but in terms of the relationship between specific genes and human development.

In this way, the clinic and the laboratory come into association in Professor Smart's natural history of Fraser syndrome, to create a space of knowledge production in human development. In these shifts between the clinical and the naturalist gaze, observing and describing the human families and mouse mutants, to the experimental mode and the construction of laboratory conditions under which experiments can take place, Professor Smart enacts key relations between clinical dysmorphology, the family and the science of growth and form and how these are helping to create not just Syndromes, but the 'new genetics'. Specifically, he is showing us how the work on the original family, and the original mouse mutants, and then the making of the mouse model, is helping them to know about the relationship of specific genes, their location on chromosomes and aspects of human development – namely that of the eyes and the kidney.

Additionally, and of equal importance, Professor Smart is not just showing me moments of translation, shifts back and forward between the laboratory and the clinic. He is illustrating how dysmorphology as a science moves from the abnormal and pathological (the genetics of the fleshy and painful problematics of Fraser syndrome), to the normal – the place of those same genes in the development of human eyes and kidneys.

Professor Smart was, as were all the expert clinical geneticists in my study, a practicing clinician, and he described many clinical cases to illustrate his practice in which he was acting as consultant to sick children and their families. And there is no doubt that his double profile as scientist and clinician are a part of the reason he was at the top of his profession and a world leader in his field.

But as we can see from his interview, as well as his role in the London Dysmorphology Club and his juxtaposition of a natural science of mouse mutants, the laboratory science and the natural history of an original clinical case, the database, the images of children and their siblings, their history and their test results, he is offering a discourse on this particular way to knowledge: a discourse not just of disease, but of the basic biology of human development.

The pathological and the normal

We are beginning to see in medical genetics, and in dysmorphology in particular, how medicine – in the context of the new genetics – is beginning to associate the pathological and the normal, in order to create new understandings about how the human organism does or does not develop.

Locating congenital abnormalities as genetic aberrations begins to institute *syndromes* as a problem of normativity in Canguilhem's (1991) sense: a problem with the organism's vitality, as its capacity to create and sustain the norms that it needs in its basic fabric to generate normal growth and form, or what Canguilhem describes as 'health' (Greco 2009). In this we can begin to see how individuals such as the mother and her daughter with Fraser syndrome are constituted in the discourse of medical genetics as both the sources and the objects/subjects of knowledge. They are the sources of knowledge because their genetic makeup is enacted as containing knowledge that produces particular healthy life forms; or, as in the case of the mother and her daughter in Professor Smart's story, do not. They become the objects of knowledge because, in revealing how their normativity does or does not work, Professor Smart and his collaborators can help discover which aspects of people's genetic makeup correlate with which aspects of the growth and form of the human organism, specifically the eye and the kidney.

This is important because, as I have discussed in Chapter 2, medicine's authority usually derives not from explicating normativity – as is frequently presumed – but from the performance of a gaze that helps make visible pathology and abnormality. As Canguilhem argues, drawing on the history of physiology and pathology in France, the pathological is never reducible to the normal. Consequently, the identification of clinical, pathological entities cannot be equated with the extension or extrapolation of the normal, either in terms of excess, or in terms of deficiency. For example, he argues that one should not confuse the *qualitative* categories of the normal with the quantitative expression of physiological values.

From Canguilhem's perspective, therefore, the pathological occupies a distinct domain of knowledge deriving from the clinic. As Greco (2009) asserts in the context of medicine, the logical priority of 'life' leads Canguilhem to insist that the difference between health and illness does not correspond in any simple way to the difference between the normal and the pathological. Being healthy involves being *normative*, rather than being *normal*. A healthy organism is a normative organism, in the sense of one (more) able to live according to its own norms of life.

But what we can learn to hear in the discourses and claims of dysmorphology is that by studying 'morphological defects' and locating their origins in genetic mutations, dysmorphology is claiming to contribute to knowledge about the normative in human development. In the alignment then of the new molecular biology, the clinic and the science of human development, medicine is extending itself as contributing to knowledge about the genetic as the source of what Foucault calls 'life itself':

> Nowadays, with the techniques at the disposal of medicine, the possibility for modifying the genetic cell structure not only affects the individual or his descendants but the entire human race. Every aspect of life now becomes the subject of medical intervention. We do not know yet whether man is capable of fabricating a living being which will make it possible to modify the entire history of life and the future of life. A new dimension of medical possibilities arises that I shall call bio-history. *The doctor and the biologist are no longer working at the level of the individual and his descendants, but are beginning to work at the level of life itself and its fundamental events.* This is a very important element in bio-history.
>
> (2004, p.11, emphasis added)

Thus, on the one hand genetic medicine's 'spirit' (Foucault 2003b, p.241) is performed as routed in a relation to a science that creates the possibility of making disease as a genetic problem visible. On the other, these relations and associations are being performed as fundamental to establishing the relationship between fleshy troubles (such as cryptopthalmus and spondactyly) and genes, as a specific *way* to knowledge, not just about disease, but about how human organisms normally grow and develop as a key aspect of their vitality.

Conclusions

In this chapter I have built on what has been discussed in earlier chapters in order to examine how various accounts of genetic medicine and dysmorphology perform in terms of medicine's dominance. This is, in part, about becoming wary of taking the conventional view of the relationship between medicine and science in the production of discoveries, as will be detailed further.

There are two important things to point out here. Firstly, the relation between science and medicine in these discourses and practices is being enacted as a site in which a specific kind of science is being accomplished and re-accomplished, one that shifts and moves back and forth between the laboratory and the clinic, the virtual and the fleshy, the engineered and the natural. In their attachment to the laboratory and to laboratory technologies, dysmorphologists enact the children and the family in these discourses as both the starting point, and the site to which genetic science returns, time and again. Within the perspective outlined we see and hear of a translational world in which, as the earlier quote from Callon put it, '*the very idea of a source or an origin point of technology is misleading because innovation is an emergent, interactive activity*' that '... involves many actors who cooperate or oppose one another' (2006, p.4, emphasis added).

The way in which Professor Smart represents the relation between medicine and science not only fits with the translation view described by Callon, discussed in Chapter 4, but appears rather strongly to *advocate* it. In this, the science being described and advocated is precisely one that shifts back and forth between the real world of bodies and families on the one hand, and on the other the laboratory as space in which to undertake experiment, and virtual technologies, such as gene mapping and the Oxford grid. Indeed, in asserting his claim in the development of the mouse model for Fraser syndrome, Professor Smart is also engaging in a new kind of medicine–science relation: one in which the transgenic mouse model itself becomes the new 'patient', and the laboratory becomes an extension of the clinic. As the clinic's extension, the laboratory is figured one moment as the site of obervations and descriptions, the next as an engineering factory where technological innovation is produced, such as mouse models, and finally as helping to progress the classification of human disease.

To return to my discussion of the place of the clinic in science, in the context of genetic knowledge, the clinical truth is being enacted in dysmorphology as both *preceding* and also as legitimating experimentation and technological innovation. And innovations must derive in the first instance from direct observation of people and their families, and in the second from observation of the transgenic mutant mouse model and its family. The engineered mutant mouse model becomes another 'real', whose organization, growth and form can be observed, and experimented with, alongside the 'visualization' of its genetic map, in ways that are according to Professor Smart, difficult to do with human families.

Additionally, I want to emphasize (ahead of a more detailed exposition in later chapters on the clinic and the family) how the medical geneticists being cited are not simply describing, but are also doing 'identity work'. Medical genetics is being enacted by dysmorphology as central to the development of the new genetics. Within these discourses and practices family and the children are rendered merely as clinical objects. In order to 'pass' in these fronts of science, the clinicians are active agents doing identity work for themselves; they present themselves as the people who are helping to push back the frontiers of the genomic unknowns in the context of the sciences of human growth and form. In this front stage of medicine's alignment of the laboratory with the clinic (along with technologies such as the Oxford grid and gene-mapping techniques, as well as animal models), the clinical gaze is enacted as if families and children are constituted as cases to be 'got'. Unsurprisingly, their humanity and sociality is effaced.

Nonetheless, as we will see when we turn to the clinic in the following two chapters, the effacement of humanity is itself partial and intermittent. What gets reinstituted in medicine's attachment to science is certainly the kind of clinical gaze that is itself a form of detachment, a detachment from the mess and flesh and pain of the field of clinical work. But it is just this doubling and shifting that I think is important: detachment in terms of the gaze masks an attachment to other allies, discourses, technologies and so forth. However, even in Professor Smart's account, the mother wrote to him directly about her daughter. The letter writing and Professor Smart's response are significant, and prompts investigation about how families attach to dysmorphologists and how dysmorphologists attach to families. As we will see when we enter the clinic, the dysmorphologists also need to immerse themselves in more everyday versions of the real – the world of bodies, persons and families – if they are to 'pass' with the family and so enable members of the family to attach to them.

Part III
Visualizing the clinic

6 Creating clinical pictures

I think we learn to be worldly from grappling with, rather than generalizing from, the ordinary. I am a creature of the mud, not the sky.

(Haraway 2007, p.3, by permission of the University of Minnesota Press)

Introduction

In the previous chapters we have seen how dysmorphologists present their work at academic and educational meetings, in published works, and in interviews. We have seen them in what I am calling, after Goffman (1980), the front stage – where they are at the blackboard, rather than in the field – presenting a highly refined picture of their clinical work. Back in the clinic, the picture is very different: here we see the organization of clinical work. Pointedly, this clinical work immerses clinicians such as Professor Smart in their 'field' of study: the bodies, homes and persons of the family. As we will see, the family here is not just made up of virtual representations of family members; it is also made up of interactions with the sentient and fleshy family.

Consequently, as I show over the next few chapters, clinical work entails 'switches' in extension as the clinicians move between engaging the family and consulting the clinical pictures that they are constructing. Some of this extension work is distributed – between nurses and doctors, in addition to family members. Critically, however, in order to muster the appropriate identities to 'pass' (Garfinkel 1967; Goffman 1980) in this field, and facilitate attachment by families, dysmorphologists must display more than the technological gaze: they must become social and human.

Arranging the clinic

In the service under study, genetic work is distributed between consultants of clinical genetics (CG), genetic specialist nurses (GSNs), other genetic associates (such as genetic counsellors), trainees in clinical genetics (specialist registrars or SpRs), other clinicians (General Practitioners and other clinical specialists) and, importantly, the family.

There is also a dedicated cytogenetic laboratory in the department, and a molecular genetics laboratory in the hospital that works closely with the department. Both these laboratories provide patient investigative services as well as homes for clinicians and scientists to work on biomedical research projects into genetic disorders. Like the clinic, then, the work of the laboratory is heterogeneous, including routine diagnostic work as well as the more heroic scientific discovery and innovation. Where tests were not available locally, clinicians could make requests for tests to other centres with expertise in the field, or seek support through the UK Genetic Testing Network, although the geneticists I spoke to stressed just how prohibitively expensive this is.

In the current service, clinical genetic process is also distributed across different occasions: the home visit, the clinical consultation and regular team meetings. After referral, but prior to most clinic appointments, the GSN or genetic counsellor makes first contact with the individual referred, called 'the proband', and their family. The proband in genetics is the initial subject of a genetic investigation that then radiates out to the family. The interesting aspect of this term is that the word is also connected to the term 'probitus' – meaning a hypothesis or argument. In this sense a proband also forms the basis of a case, in both senses of the word: as well as the subject becoming a medical case, it is also the starting point for the construction of an argument on which a diagnosis is grounded.

Many families receive a home visit prior to their clinic appointment, the purpose of which is to 'take a history', create a family tree, and collect relevant materials (e.g. photographs). In addition to the different 'histories', the nurse obtains permission to trace and acquire medical records for relevant family members, including test results and autopsy reports, which will be used in the creation of the child's 'medical pedigree'. A report of this visit, including the family tree, is placed in the medical records held by the clinical genetic service. It is then discussed at the clinical team meeting, often prior to the family's visit to the clinic.

Some weeks or months after this initial work, the child and other family members come to the clinic for a consultation. Timing here relates to how interesting or urgent the team assesses the case to be. Usually, both the consultant and the GSN who has conducted the home visit are present at the initial clinical consultation. Here, the consultant discusses the route of referral and the family tree assembled by the nurse, and looks at test results and scans. They also do their own history and conduct a clinical examination. They do this by asking the parents or the proband themselves a series of questions in a pretty routine format – about the pregnancy, the child's development and their health, as well as about other members of the family and their health and development. Either simultaneously or in between taking this history, the doctor will ask for the child to undress or to be undressed, and examine the child.

A typical dysmorphology examination 'starts from the top' (consultant dysmorphologist, field notes, clinical consultation with the patient, Sheila). Generally, the clinical geneticist carefully inspects the head, the face, the tongue, hands, trunk and back, joints, feet. Measurements of head circumference, height and weight are also taken. The clinician is looking at the shape, size and position of features. The doctor may look closely at specific aspects that arise as the examination unfolds – such as neurological reflexes or genitalia or in the eyes. They may also take photographs of those features that appear distinctive as well as examine photographs of other family members.

Potential diagnoses, tests and other materials that may be required to aid a diagnosis are sometimes discussed. More rarely, the causes of the condition, its progression and the risk of recurrence are also discussed where these have been more established. Many of the consultants that I interviewed also told me that they did a lot of what some of them called 'homework' in between each formal element of the diagnostic process. This included searching databases, discussing descriptions of cases with colleagues across the world via email, and seeking out and reading up on articles with similar descriptions.

All these facets of clinical work are used to build a 'clinical picture' of the child and their family. This clinical picture is regularly reviewed at weekly team meetings. The team meetings observed during fieldwork usually consisted of all members of the clinical team, namely the special registrars and one or two genetic specialist nurses, working under the direction of the genetic consultant. In these meetings members review and prioritize new referrals, construct a diagnosis for both new and ongoing cases, gather materials to aid diagnosis and organize future clinics. They often do this while looking at slides of the photographs of children and their relations assembled during the clinical process.

Clinical technologies

As well as all the usual clinical technologies and processes, such as clinical history, biochemistry and CT scans, there are two distinctive clinic-based technologies used in dysmorphology diagnosis: photographs and family trees. These are described in turn in the next few sections.

The clinical team uses two types of photograph: those taken during the clinical consultation, and family photographs collected by the GSN at the initial home visit or brought to the clinic by the family. Photographs taken in the clinic are used to make a record of specific and 'unusual' features, such as unusual hands and feet or a 'distinctive' face. Throughout the book I illustrate the text with these two types of photographs.

At team meetings the photographs, reproduced as slides, are projected onto a screen and discussed. Family photographs are used to trace specific features, either in the proband themselves or across other family members. The most relevant of these photographs are filed in the medical records.

As we have seen in Chapter 3, it is these photographs (rather than the patients themselves) which are subsequently circulated at clinical meetings of experts at regional, national and international levels for teaching, research and diagnostic purposes[1] as well as in published academic papers. I offer an in-depth analysis of the photographs and their use in Chapters 6 and 7.

The second technology, the family tree, is composed initially by the GSN during the home visit. Turning the family tree into a medical pedigree is a mundane practice that, through processes of inclusion and exclusion, begins to construct patterns and relations between bodies, persons, health and ideas of inheritance. Representational conventions with which to construct these pedigrees in genetic medicine are examined in various other contexts (e.g. Gibbon 2002; Nukaga and Cambrosio 1997).

How the process of making medical pedigrees constructs family and kinship has been described elsewhere (Atkinson *et al.* 2001). Others have noted how the family tree draws on wider cultural constructions of bloodlines, breeding and inheritance in constructing biological relatedness (Bouquet 1994).

It it is important to see that the medical pedigree does not merely report or 'picture' family relations, but that it is one of the key mechanisms whereby such relations – and indeed families themselves – are actively produced. It is also where biological, as opposed to social, closeness is being reinstated, with the effect of medicalizing reproduction and legitimating clinical access to the family. Pressing these matters in the rest of this chapter, as well as the chapters that follow, will help show how clinical genetics gets 'inside' the family and turns family members into allies.

Reproducing the biological family

To give some idea of how the creation of the family tree as the technology that reproduces biological family is related to the initial home visit, I have included the following extract from the opening of the GSN's visit to the home of George and his family:

[Arrive with Susan (the GSN) at a large, detached post-war house with large iron gates and a short drive that leads up to a large porch. Greeted by the parents, both in their mid to late 30s. Don't see their two children, hear them playing upstairs. Taken through to a large sitting room by the mother while the father goes to make tea – he brings through a tray later in the meeting. Susan sits on the sofa, George's mother sits close to her side, the father when he joins the meeting stands a little apart, leaning against a piece of furniture near the fireplace.]

SUSAN (GSN): We had a letter from Dr Bond [paediatrician]. This [the visit] is to ask you a little bit more information and what you expect to get out of it, explain about Dr White [the consultant geneticist to whom George has been referred], who she is, when her clinic is and when the best day is and just go through things a little bit with George [son]. I'll take a family tree [she opens out her file and takes a sheet and starts to record the family history].

Susan arrives and enters the house and sits on the sofa. The greeting and the making of the tea signal the sociality of the occasion. As a GSN, she explains to George's mother why she is there, and opens up her file, announcing the business of the visit, which is to give information about the clinic, to take a history and 'take' a family tree.

However, the first thing to note is how clinical genetics penetrates the home and the private space of the family. Clinicians account for this visit in terms of helping the families to feel at ease with their visit to the clinic. But this visit also helps ground the clinical work in the material and semiotic space of the contemporary family home.

Surveillance in the home

When they report back to the team, it emerges that the nurses who do these visits are also making an assessment of the family: they notice things and make a reading of the family from the state of the home, particularly in terms of order and disorder, and from how parents and other members relate to each other – how they look or conduct themselves. This kind of surveillance work is quite normal in child and reproductive health care, for example when midwives and health visitors make home visits during and after pregnancy (e.g. Bloor and Mackintosh 1990). Many comments made by the nurses at team meetings indicate that this is a part of what they are doing, such as 'there was an old fridge in the front garden', or 'Mum is obviously delayed', or 'they are clearly not coping'.

In the following part of Susan's visit she is taking the family history as the basis for making a family tree:

GEORGE'S MOTHER: My husband is adopted.
SUSAN: That will be a short side! Does he know anything about his family?
GEORGE'S MOTHER: Just that they're Polish.
SUSAN: [Begins to take a family tree, husband's and mother's names and dates of birth then] How many children do you have?
GEORGE'S MOTHER: George and Jacob.
SUSAN: The dates of birth for both?
GEORGE'S MOTHER: George 1987 and Jacob 2001.
SUSAN: Any other pregnancies?
GEORGE'S MOTHER: No.
SUSAN: Any health problems?
GEORGE'S MOTHER: No.
SUSAN: Pregnancies fine?
GEORGE'S MOTHER: Yes.

The session begins with George's mother proffering the information that the father is adopted and Susan checks if he knows anything about his family; the mother says only that they are Polish. Susan makes a joke – 'That will be a short side!' Susan then begins the question and answer session – closed questions about the father, the mother and their children. She also asks about the pregnancy and whether the mother has any health problems. In this way she draws George's mother into the correlation between health, family, pregnancy and reproduction.

Susan goes on to extend this questioning out from the nuclear family to previous generations (George's mother's parents and grandparents) and across generations, to her siblings and their children, thus bringing the 'extended' family into view:

SUSAN: Your brothers and sisters?
GEORGE'S MOTHER: A__ 40 years old, E__ 39.
SUSAN: Any children?
GEORGE'S MOTHER: A__ has 3 children, L__, M__ and J__; E__ has a baby boy.
SUSAN: Are they all fit and well as far as you know?
GEORGE'S MOTHER: Yes, J__ has had some speech therapy but he's fine now.
SUSAN: Did your mother have any miscarriages?
GEORGE'S MOTHER: No.
SUSAN: Your parents are fit and well and fine?
GEORGE'S MOTHER: Yes, although father has cancer.
SUSAN: How old is he now?
GEORGE'S MOTHER: 76.
SUSAN: Is he local?
GEORGE'S MOTHER: They live locally in ____.
SUSAN: How are they coping?
GEORGE'S MOTHER: I get up as much as I can but work [she is a doctor] gets in the way.
SUSAN: Are you full time?
GEORGE'S MOTHER: Yes.
SUSAN: So your mother's fine but exhausted, and her siblings?
GEORGE'S MOTHER: Her sister died in 2000 in her 70s, a brother and two sisters.
SUSAN: Any problems with their children or their development?
GEORGE'S MOTHER: C__ [mother's brother's son] is a bit odd, we think it's more of the upbringing rather than anything else, he's a bit slow, but from family talk it sounded as though he was a bit under-stimulated as a child. So environment.
SUSAN: How old is he?
GEORGE'S MOTHER: Late 30s.
SUSAN: Does he work?
GEORGE'S MOTHER: Yes but he lives at home, he has no independent life.
SUSAN: Was he a bit slow at school?
GEORGE'S MOTHER: It's a bit difficult because we moved away. Uncle P__ had 3 children, they are all fine, but uncle T__, he didn't achieve what the girls did.
SUSAN: Grandparents?
GEORGE'S MOTHER: They are fine, grandfather was diabetic, he died when he was 72, grandmother was strong as an ox, she was 75 when she died but no chronic health problems.
SUSAN: How old is your mother now?

In this phase of the questioning Susan moves between eliciting factual information about health, age and longevity, and more qualitative questions about whether

George's mother's parents are coping or not, and whether there were any problems with health or development in the children across her parents' and grandparents' generations. George's mother proffers observations and assessments here: that her uncle's son was a bit odd, a bit slow, but attributes this to 'upbringing' and sums up that, from family talk, he was 'understimulated': she summarizes by attributing the problems with this child to environment – i.e. as nothing inherent.

George's mother then goes on to offer some unsolicited information, as if the question and answer session has got her to reconsider her family's birth and reproductive history, to remember something that is not simply a part of well-rehearsed family talk:

GEORGE'S MOTHER: 66. The only thing is my grandmother did have a stillborn little boy, it was 'termish' [nearly went to full term] and he was buried, so at that time it must have been full term. Gran had just him and the four that lived. My mother was a W____ [surname] [she goes into details of the family history], mother was from 'a well to do family', 'landed', 'she traded down'. You know, family secrets, there was a half brother, he's dead but his children are fine. The son had three, the daughter two, they're fine, though my sister, says L__, there is something not quite right, she's very shy and uncommunicative and as we get older, my sister thought she had a weird syndrome, she thought one of those X things, she's little.
SUSAN: Is she noticeably short?
GEORGE'S MOTHER: No.
SUSAN: Any other features?
GEORGE'S MOTHER: Not really, not that I can put a finger on.
SUSAN: How old is her mum?
GEORGE'S MOTHER: About 40.
SUSAN: L__ had no children?
GEORGE'S MOTHER: Yes.
SUSAN: Did she do OK at school?
GEORGE'S MOTHER: Yes, but I think it was hidden because she was overactive, L__ is ferociously bright but with all the problems that go with that, she never really settled.
SUSAN: What about your father's parents?

George's mother offers a description and account of her grandmother's stillborn child that was 'termish' and then gives a little social history of how her mother had 'traded down' in her marriage. She then mentions there was a half brother [to her mother], a family secret, but that his children are fine, except for one grandchild, whom George's mother's sister thought might have one of those 'weird syndromes': she's ferociously bright, shy, uncommunicative and short. Thus the taking of the family tree incites the mother to juxtapose the social history of the family, including its secrets and darker markings, with its reproductive and health history.

In summary, Susan asks George's mother to provide information about her blood relations and her relations by marriage across four generations: grandparents, parents, herself and her siblings and their children. George's mother willingly describes and accounts for each in terms of their health and anything 'unusual'.

Parents readily engage with tracing the family history, and assessing not just the health but also the behaviour and development of family members, including their own, as well as revealing family secrets and characterizations – such as being the 'black sheep', or the existence of mysterious half brothers and sisters. George's mother proffers her own and her sister's assessment of other relations as maybe having a 'weird syndrome'. This is not just because George's mother is a doctor: many families engage in this kind of assessment and evaluation of their relations (see also Featherstone *et al.* 2006).

What we can see from this exchange is that Susan is not just eliciting a *medical* pedigree by 'taking a clinical history'. Rather the note taking and chart making is inciting discussion and description of family members *by family members*. The importance of legitimating this kind of discussion – in terms of how they look and why their social and personal histories matter – is now discussed.

Exercising the parents

This first part of the home visit is all about focussing on biological kin, which has the effect of bringing family members into relatedness in very specific ways, what anthropologists sometimes refer to as 'kinning' (Howell 2006). In so doing the nurse co-creates with the family its shape and form, represented by a hand-written family tree. George's mother, like many parents, participates in connecting ideas of relatedness (biological and by marriage), reproduction and 'deformations' in terms of strange children or mysterious illnesses and deaths. She points to those areas of family that are difficult to illuminate – because of deaths and secrets.

After the extracts above Susan goes on to explore George's father's health and development, the pregnancy and birth of George, and then they turn to George's history – how he has developed, how he looks and what the parents noticed about him and when. There is a problem here for Nurse Susan in doing a full medical pedigree because George's father is adopted and there is no medical or developmental history of his biological parents or siblings – this may be why he stands at the fireplace for the first part of the session, because he feels excluded as someone not related by biological ties.

The shape and form of George's family is thus asymmetrical: a further deformation and one leg of the tree will be absent, like an amputation or what Goffman refers to as an 'abomination' of the body (1963, p.4). But note how the abomination here is in the shape and form of the family, not any one person.

Observation of these interactions, and subsequent comments at team meetings, suggest that the nurse is making an informal assessment of the family in various terms, such as their 'commitment' to getting a diagnosis (see also White *et al.* 2012), individual and family 'capacity' (intellectual, [dys]functional), as well as 'family' and 'social' dynamics, for example in terms of how they are 'coping'. Here, when presenting the family at a team meeting, mothers and/or fathers can be described as 'delayed', or as not quite 'coping'.

I want to emphasize how the interactions over, as well as the materiality of constructing, a family tree begin to *exercise* parents in making correlations: between family histories, how people look, their health and how they cope, their behaviour, with reproduction and biological relatedness. Thus family relatedness, and specifically relations of reproduction, are being enacted in very particular ways through these encounters: as correlated with health and ill health and the kinds of persons (intellectual, social and behavioural), that families create. And family members, especially parents, are being engaged to participate in these enactments.

Critically, it must be remembered that the implicit purpose of these encounters is to search for the origins of problems in the child, such as George. And in this case there are all kinds of undercurrents and traces subtlety being surfaced, particularly where the history is slightly problematic (secrets, trading-down, adoptions and unknown others). Thus, in the history of the mother's family, but also in the absence of a history of the father's family, there is a search for anything unusual in the family that might be at the root of George's problems: if there is nothing in the mother's family, then maybe it is the adopted father and his unknown family, that are 'to blame'? At this stage there is no clinical examination of the child.

As well as noting how referral of a person for a genetic consultation opens up the genetic clinic's access to the family and to the home, it is important to emphasize how family is participant in this opening up. As already mentioned, one of the things being gauged at the home visit is the family's commitment and capacity to participate in the long and arduous process of genetic diagnosis (see also White *et al.* 2012). The family tree engages family in the construction of the family's formation, and associates issues of health, illness, and deformity to the form of the family. I shall return to these relationships in depth in later chapters on the family.

Compiling the family tree

A family tree thus begins to be compiled from the initial home visit, and grows from there into what becomes a medical pedigree. Each stage in this transformation becomes a part of the case notes. By the time it becomes a medical pedigree each member of the kindred is represented by a symbol to indicate their gender and latent or manifest disease status if known, along with details of their name, age, pregnancy history, health status and any other potentially relevant information. The medical pedigree serves as a much sanitized visual representation of family relationships that includes medical conditions, and may also eventually as it is built over time, contain any genetic diagnosis or positive tests results, including carrier status (see Figure 6.1).

Specifically, the family tree takes on a life of its own: its fabricated nature is effaced and it is, like other clinical materials, placed in the proband's medical

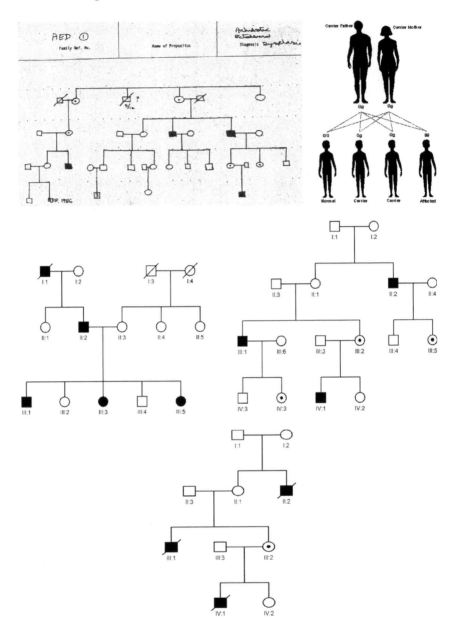

Figure 6.1 The growth of a family tree into a medical pedigree: from the handwritten notes through to the formalized medical pedigree. Reproduced with kind permission of Angus Clarke.

records as a representation of the family (cf. Gibbon 2002). So the construction of a family tree allows the clinical team to map similarities in diseases, as well as in features, across family members who are biologically related, or related by marriage. However, the visual representation of the family tree does not contain any of the 'extra' contextualizing descriptions of family by the nurse or by family members of themselves and their relations that help ground the clinical picture. These aspects may or may not be retained in the memories of the team, but they are erased in the documentation.

We can see from this analysis that the clinic in dysmorphology does not only concern itself with the individual – with the molar, the organism as a singular entity – but with the family, and with the family *as an extended bodily form* made up of connected parts, a figure that becomes sedimented in the form of the family tree.

Through a process of inscription, the family tree, together with the photographs, begin to connect and mark some features and 'bodily troubles' as possibly familial and/or inherited. Other features drop out of sight. What is traced and simultaneously 'erased' (Derrida 1978) is the interactive work through which families create their own descriptions and the nurse takes impressions of families as social as well as biological phenomena. These aspects, like the soil, mulch, water and light, which enable trees to grow, leave their traces in the clinical interpretation of a family's troubles, but they gradually get translated, sanitized and their origins erased from any record of the case.

Doing dysmorphology

Clinical genetics thus draws upon several clinic-based technologies in the work of categorizing patients. Photographs and family trees are among the material resources for clinical genetic knowledge practices, and help us to understand how patients are categorized. And, as has been seen in previous chapters, dysmorphology also draws at moments upon various techniques of chromosome and molecular analysis.

Although most dysmorphic syndromes are thought to involve submicroscopic genetic mutations, and changes in DNA sequence, for many syndromes there are not yet any specific tests. Even when a relevant test exists, it does not necessarily determine the diagnostic categorization. Instead, what gets enacted by dysmorphology practice is that it is the gaze of the clinic that can *read* both the fleshy family as well as virtual representations of bodies and faces of a child and their family for their signs.

Further, while dysmorphology discourse and practice enact the gaze of the clinician as able to read the bodies and faces of a child and their family, the gaze emerges not just as monolithic, inculcated in medical schools and acculturated on occasions such as Dysmorphology Club. Rather, for their gaze to 'pass' (Garfinkel 1967; Goffman 1980) their different audiences, clinicians have to be *motile*. They do not only have to be passed by fellow scientists and clinicians in the academy, such as we have seen at Dysmorphology Club. To gain access to the family, and enable immersion in the field, the clinician also has *to pass* with the family, as a fellow human.

We can hear some of this complexity in the description of practice by Professor Fox, a world-leading expert and mother of UK Dysmorphology:

> I love the science, but it is the clinic that matters ... I do my own history and examination. As I take a history I read the family – what do they want? What have they noticed? And I watch the child. I do the examination sitting the child on my lap – 'ooh it's hot in here, Daddy do you want to take your coat off?' I look at the faces. Hold up bangles – give the child one, then the other – they know I am nice. But I am looking at palm creases, motor function, little fingers, toes, eye movements – hold the bangle up and look at eye movements. I am looking for anomalies, differences, patterns. The family tree helps me get a feel for the family – and for patterns across the family. I'm very visual. I take my own photos – photos are a part of the clinical notes – *but a special face marks them as a problem.*
>
> (Author interview, 2003–2004)

Professor Fox is the person who I described in Chapter 2 as working alongside Professor Smart at the London Dysmorphology Club meeting, schooling neophytes in the art of seeing syndromes. In this interview of almost two hours, she spoke to me with her eyes closed, smiling, grimacing, frowning, as she remembered each family she had worked closely with. She exuded carefulness, exactness, curiosity, as well as real attachment to the families and her stories of them.

Professor Fox describes herself as interacting with the family where she can examine the child's response, their 'behaviour', and the form of their body (e.g. palm creases), as at the same time she has to 'pass' (Garfinkel 1967; Goffman 1980) with the child and the family as human: sitting the child on her lap, persuading the child to be helped off with their clothes, holding up bangles. She figures herself as clever, humorous and devious, stressing the undercover watchfulness and observation – ' ... they know I am nice. But I am looking at palm creases ... hold up the bangle and look at eye movements.'

We can hear in her discourse how dysmorphology focuses on shape and form, and the appearance as well as the function of bodies and their parts: 'I look at the faces'. While we have seen how nurses at the home visit help construct a family tree by taking a history, Professor Fox, like many of the clinicians interviewed and observed, emphasizes how 'I do my own history': but, as she 'takes the history' she 'reads the family'. This involves picking up on what the family themselves have noticed so that the family becomes the extension of her gaze; they are her eyes and ears for what they can see and she cannot (as of yet).

Professor Fox describes herself as doing this work of observing in the context of a *process*: she is making a reading and 'getting a feel' through intense processes of crosschecking and contextualization. Yet she is doing all this in a way that still makes her acceptable to the parents and the child. All the observations of geneticists at work in the clinic conveyed these same kinds of careful practices and processes, revealing a kind of attachment to the fleshy family, not just the virtual family represented by photographs, charts or test results.

Immersion in the family

The attachment to the fleshy family is much more then than just 'sentimental work' (Featherstone *et al.* 2006). Rather, like Hercule Poirot, or traditional ethnographers for that matter, the clinicians are insisting on a particular kind of immersed, or 'situated' (Clarke, 2005) knowledge practice: one which is much more closely aligned to humanist representations of clinical practice (see also Greco 2009).

Clinicians extend this insistence to representations of the family. For example, in the following extract, the doctor insists on making her own readings, looking for herself, not just at reports produced by others:

> And people from outside they don't understand why I should want to look at the scan. Not just – they don't understand why the report's not sufficient. But it doesn't give you, you don't see the pattern and the pattern is. Well it's like doing dysmorphology without seeing the child and without a picture. It's the same thing. It's exactly the same thing. And it doesn't mean other people are wrong. I mean, they often think I want to see it because I want to prove them wrong. It's got nothing to do with that. But I've got my own picture and this is the way I understand the world if you like. In a sense. That's the thing about dysmorphology as well, this is the way you understand what you are doing and I understand the world by looking, by seeing.
>
> (Author interview with Dr Fellows, 2nd generation dysmorphologist, 2003–2004)

In this extract Dr Fellows, like many of her colleagues, stresses the need to look at the real thing – whether it be a scan or the child and their family – in order to be able to see. But 'looking' is situated; it includes, as I have shown earlier, dysmorphologists doing their own questioning over the exact history of the proband's case – both in terms of pregnancy and the birth, as well as in terms of the history of the child since birth.

Thus, looking and seeing are not quite the same things. Seeing is what happens after looking; it is enacted by dysmorphologists as the effect of gaze as an act of interpretation or even by some as innate, a 'gift' – Professor Smart in Chapter 3 said it was genetic! But, as we have heard in Professor Fox's and Dr Fellows's discourses, looking involves immersion in the real world. This in turn means both attaching to family and passing as a fellow human.

Like Drs Fox and Fellows in the extracts above, dysmorphologists emphasize that a critical aspect of their work is *seeing the face as unusual* because it is this, together with pattern recognition that can indicate the presence of a syndrome. Some syndromes have a typical face, but there may be 'variability of expression', so that the syndrome may be clearly or mildly expressed (see also Selicorni *et al.* 2007). This term 'expressed' is a common feature of the geneticists' world – it refers to how the phenotype is an expression of the genotype. The face then, in this discursive domain, becomes a 'text' written strongly or mildly by the syndrome.

The art of recognition

Where the syndrome is clearly 'expressed', there may be what dysmorphologists call a 'gestalt moment' of instant recognition, such as that described by Professor Smart in his account of the woman and her daughter with Fraser syndrome in Chapter 4: the moment he saw her in the clinic he says that he knew what he was looking at.

This is not always the case, and the face of the child may need to be set explicitly in a broader context:

> The combination of specific and typical dysmorphisms can sometimes give an overall impression of a facial appearance at a glance ('gestalt') which can be the key clue in getting immediately to a diagnosis (for example, Down syndrome). If a diagnosis is not made straight away, it is then important to focus on each single facial trait and to compare them with other family members' ones (siblings and parents), in order to determine whether the features noted are familial or not, and therefore be much more related to a syndromic pattern.
>
> (Winter 1996, p.125)

In this extract we are given some idea then of what is meant by reading the family, and why, as Professor Fox emphasizes in her interview with me, they need to look at the faces of the family. Unless the diagnosis is 'immediate' – 'at a glance' – then it is important to focus on each single facial trait, and compare faces across family members to see if features are familial or not.

What is being enacted here – either way – is an idea of a special gaze. Sometimes this is enacted as instantaneous, at other times as requiring explicit contextualization and cross-checking. Of course as we have already noted, the first time a clinician sees a child their gaze may have already been situated – at the team meeting in discussion of the referral, and by the nurse in her report of the home visit. Either way, the clinicians are enacting a gaze that can 'see by looking'.

It is seeing a syndromic pattern in the features of family faces that dysmorphologists say they can read by looking. This is a vital aspect of their expertise, sometimes it is instantaneous, but more often than not they enact it as part of a long process grounded in the family, requiring many cross-checks, especially involving looking across the family as well as other reported cases. They describe this as 'pattern recognition'. For example, another dysmorphologist, Dr Albert, told me a story in his interview about a very sick newborn infant who was referred to him. On his first visit to the baby in intensive care he could not see anything particularly dysmorphic in the face of the baby, but then on the next visit to the baby he met the mother and he could see the syndrome in the face of the mother. He reported that the likeness between the mother and child helped him identify what was wrong with the baby.

Dysmorphologists also say how they follow up 'feelings' or hunches from looking at the face of a child, first by looking at the family but also by trying to find 'handles':

> ... if I think the face is unusual, you've obviously got to look at the parents to see if there is a likeness or whatever. If you can't make a gestalt diagnosis, don't recognize the face, and the chromosomes are normal, then these days you wonder about doing more specific or detailed chromosome tests. There is rather a vague concept that that child looks a bit chromosomal – sort of thing. Which is kind of just a feeling that there is something about the faces of some children with bits missing from their chromosomes, that you just have to look, if you know what I mean ... We don't [always] do them – chromosomes – we do them on the ones that look chromosomal basically. So we might use that approach. Otherwise we are going – if we haven't got any gestalt – and the chromosome test doesn't work, then we're stuck. The other thing we might do is, we might, if the child has a small head for example, we might have a brain scan, a CT or MRI scan, and we might consider that – that might give us a specific handle; or then – if it is a child – order a skeletal survey, that might give us more of a handle on what the bones look like. So there are other handles if you don't get clinical [recognition], further tests.
>
> (Author interview with Dr Godfrey, 2003–2004, a second generation dysmorphologist, who said he had 'come through' Professor Smart)

Critically, this discipline is about being able to see something in children and/or family members as dysmorphic, or malformed, but also to see that these malformations are produced because of something wrong at the levels of chromosomes and genes.

This for dysmorphologists is 'looking a bit chromosomal'. Some experts argue that this malformation has to be visible in the face of the child and/or their kin, while others take the view that it can include any feature across the bodies of children and their kin, including as Dr Fellows suggested, their behaviour. Ordinarily, however, the doctors stressed that an individual or their kin has to look dysmorphic, and that clinicians have to be able to see this look.

Embodying the gaze

All the experts observed or interviewed emphasized that they belonged to the school in which this gaze had to be embodied by the clinician: it could not be programmed into a computer. Indeed, some stressed that there are computer programs being developed and standardized measures of facial features being incorporated into the assessment of dysmorphia, although they thought these would be useful, at most, merely as cross-checks on their own perception.

This resistance amongst the British dysmorphologists that I followed was in the face of pressure to make the gaze 'more objective'. For example, Loos *et al.* (2003) reported on a research project on development of computer recognition tools for dysmorphic faces. The tools were tested against clinicians, with the clinicians being reported as not being as good as the computer tool at recognizing dysmorphia. Computerized images are also used to create simulation programs through which the photos of children can be matched with the image of a syndrome (Clarke, undated).

There is some controversy, even dispute, between dysmorphologists regarding this issue. The computer simulation of faces relies upon stabilized classification of dysmorphic syndromes as present in an individual, whose face can be measured and held against the face of a 'representative subject'. In contrast, the experts I interviewed said that they had been trained in a different tradition, by the mother and father of dysmorphology Professor Fox and Professor Smart, and that because children change over time and because of the problem of racial and other kinds of variability, standardized measurements and programs were not very useful.

In addition, when we enter the clinic and examine how dysmorphologists do their work, we can see that they are not just looking at a face, they are looking *across* faces, bodies, and other representations of family members, including their medical, social and pregnancy histories. Dysmorphologists are building a clinical picture, not just of a child, but of the child and their relations.

As is discussed in greater detail in the rest of this chapter, there is considerable motility as to how the recognition of dysmorphia is enacted on the ground. At one moment the dysmorphology gaze is enacted as if it is embodied in an individual – the sovereign subject of a clinical gaze. In the next, the work of establishing the presence or absence of dysmorphia is enacted as belonging to a collective enterprise.

Seeing dysmorphia

Fitting someone's features into a classification of dysmorphia is enacted as not in any way self-evident; it has to be established. As Latour (1987, p.12) puts it, the classification has to be made to 'hold'. This is where we see the clinic most clearly enacted as a *centre of discretion*, made up of sovereign subjects who can agree or disagree with each other's 'opinions'.

We have heard already that photographs of children and family members are key materials. Specifically, at clinical team meetings photographs are passed around, and each member looks for distinctive physical signs and indicators on the body of the child and their kin. In the following extract, the team is examining photographs of Sam:

LOTTIE (GSN): A follow-up. [Adds that she and the SpR had seen Sam previously at the clinic.]

DR BYTHE (SPR): Not particularly dysmorphic.
DR WHITE (CG): Coarse looking though.

The team offer their observations of how Sam looks to them. Although Dr Bythe describes Sam as 'not particularly dysmorphic', the consultant notes that he is 'coarse looking' and this subtle distinction helps keep Sam within the realm of dysmorphology. It is important to remember here that dysmorphia is categorized as a feature of how someone looks that is not necessarily abnormal, but has a distinctive quality to it, which in this case is 'coarseness'.

A common question raised while looking at the photographs is whether a patient looks dysmorphic *enough*. Consider the following discussion about Charles:

LOTTIE (GSN): Yes, he's the new one to be seen, query Sotos [She brings out two family photographs from her file. The first is of a young man in his late teens standing in a bathroom doorway with a towel wrapped around his waist – it looks as though he has just got out of the bath. In the second photograph he is sitting with his twin sister in either a restaurant or a bar, they are both smiling into the camera. The photographs are passed around and examined by all the members of the team.] He's got learning difficulties.
SARAH (GSN): [Looking at photos] They're [his features] not striking. There were no complications during his birth.
DR LITTLE (CG): [He places the photographs back in the envelope and reads from the notes, commenting that his birth-weight was low even for a twin. The consultant then takes the photographs out of the envelope again, scrutinizes them and passes them to the specialist registrar.] I'm hopeless at talking about what I see, he has got a high forehead – but [gesturing to Charles's eyes] they're not down-slanting.
SARAH: Apart from his forehead he doesn't look dysmorphic enough.
DR LITTLE: But the forehead is quite striking.
LOTTIE: His CT [brain] scan was normal.
[They go on to speculate about other possible genetic origins to Charles's problems.]

As the various members of the team scrutinize the photographs, they are considering whether Charles does or does not fit a diagnostic category, Sotos syndrome. Figure 6.2 shows a photo of a child diagnosed with Sotos syndrome taken from an article in the *Journal of Medical Genetics* (Robertson and Bankier 1999). As we can see from the extract above, Charles is not self-evidently a representative subject of Sotos in the clinic. Rather, slides of Charles are juxtaposed with those of his twin sister to see if Charles's face has the look of Sotos rather than sharing a similar look with his sister, who does not have the same problems as Charles.

The initial gaze of the clinical team is further contextualised by the nurse, Lottie, who, presumably drawing on her history of the family from her home visit, points out that Charles has learning difficulties. The second nurse, Sarah,

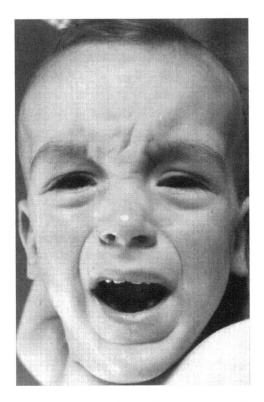

Figure 6.2 Typical features of Sotos syndrome. Reproduced with kind permission of the BMJ Publishing Group Ltd.

sums up Charles's look, stating that his features are 'not striking', but maintains ambiguity over Charles's diagnosis by reminding the team that his learning difficulties were not caused by complications at birth (e.g. anoxia).

Dr Little also hesitates, suggesting that Charles's birth-weight was too low for him to have Sotos syndrome. As he puts the photographs of Charles and his sister away, Dr Little seems to be about to dispose of Charles, relegating him, as it were, to the realm of normality. However, in drawing the photographs back out of the envelope, he draws Charles back into the clinic.

Making it genetic

Dr Little legitimates his action by stating that it is his inability to articulate what he sees that is the problem, rather than the absence of something to see. Even though the second nurse suggests that Charles 'doesn't look dysmorphic enough', Dr Little persists by stating that the forehead is 'quite striking'. Here he is enacting a sovereign gaze: he is the subject that can see 'the real'; he just lacks the words to express what this might be.

Sarah appears to reinforce Lottie's pressure to move Charles out of the clinic by saying his CT scan was normal. However, the ambiguity and undecidability over whether Charles is dysmorphic enough, together with his learning difficulties, is enough to keep Charles in the clinic, and the team continuing the search for genetic explanations for Charles's troubles.

This is the gaze, the gaze that is claiming to see dysmorphia, although it is a kind of seeing that is explicitly contextualized through the processes of the clinic, such as by recalling the history, and by examining photos of the sister.

Thus a look may be made to gain in significance through being juxtaposed with other observations. For example, in another case, Louise, it is her 'small jaw' that becomes significant in the context of other observations: a cleft palate and a heart defect. Similarly, Charles's 'striking' forehead when juxtaposed with his learning difficulties is suggestive of a pathology, even though the nurses do not consider that he looks sufficiently dysmorphic.

The signs across different systems (long limbs, low brow, down-slanting eyes, pointy chin, hearing difficulties) can be made visible as abnormalities because there are the beginnings of a system (however incomplete) with which to trace and link them. Therefore, the significance of any distinctive feature is constituted by the presence of other signs across different systems. *Or not.* The identification of the presence (or absence) of the pathological is being enacted as a matter of clinical discretion. What is always held in play is that discretion enacts the possibility of deferral.

That is, even when one feature is defined as dysmorphic, this description is still indeterminate. Fixing a patient within a categorization depends upon the skill/craft of the clinical team to see other effects in a patient's history that are either associated with a known syndrome or that seem 'syndromic', that is, suggestive of a syndrome. For example, in the extract below, the team describes a referral, a young woman, Fiona, with a 'pointy chin':

DR SMITH (CG): 16 [years old].
SARAH (GSN): What is it?
DR SMITH: Slightly unusual face, pointy chin. Didn't identify a syndrome. Learning difficulties, not major though. She's had facial surgery.

Even though her features do not fit neatly into any established category, so that she is not 'a major', Fiona's physical features, in conjunction with the evidence that she has learning difficulties, are enough to keep her within the clinic.

Seeing a patient as dysmorphic, and therefore potentially syndromic, is therefore a matter of juxtaposing a patient's 'unusual' visible features with their other problems such as 'learning difficulties'. The features partly take on their significance as dysmorphic because they are unusual in themselves, and partly through their association with other problems.

At this stage, there is also the requirement, as I have already shown in the discussion about Charles, to differentiate between genetic and other possible origins of dysmorphia and learning difficulties, such as anoxia at birth or foetal alcohol syndrome. The origin of features still has to be accomplished and be made visible. Here, it is important to differentiate between demonstrating that the patient's features are familial or indicative of a syndrome, and as having a genetic base that is or is not inherited. For clinicians, such as those talking in the extract above, this requires them to see the bodies of babies and children in terms of how they have developed from their conception to the moment they encounter them in the clinic.

The critical question that dysmorphologist's practices begin to raise is whether the abnormalities in the growth and form of a child represent a failure of reproduction or an aberration at the genetic level. As will be seen, this is not just important in terms of counselling the family over future reproductive plans or in terms of an individual's prognosis, as important as these things are to the clinic. Rather, it is also enacted as important in terms of building knowledge about the genotype and its expression.

Making it familial

Making it familial relies on the established clinical skill of seeing patterns of inheritance across generations. To do this, the clinical team draw together three strands of clinical (not laboratory-based) evidence: the family tree, accounts of the proband's medical history and clinical examination, and family photographs described above. Seeing features and other effects, such as learning difficulties across 'the family', helps strengthen the evidence that the patient's features are genetic. However, not all inherited features or traits are the effects of an underlying syndrome and part of the clinical work is to distinguish between what is familial, and what is (possibly) syndromic.

Where photographic evidence is available, the physical features of family members are examined, discussed and compared. In the following extract, the team discusses Anna, a new referral, and her family:

SARAH (GSN): [Sally brings out a small, laminated, professional school photograph of Anna as a young girl from her file. In the photograph with her are her three younger siblings in a row, arranged in age order – eldest to youngest. She passes this to Consultant 1, who studies it closely.] They all need to be seen in clinic [she reels off a list of developmental and behavioural problems that the children have]. Three have learning difficulties, one attends a special school.

DR LITTLE (CG): [After studying the photograph for some time.] Two have 'big heads'. [He points this out to the researcher.]

SARAH: They had CT scans, which failed to show anything up.

[They all agree that they need to start by looking at Anna.]

Family photographs and family histories allow the team to look for features across family members. In discussing the case of Anna, the team traces features such as 'big heads' and learning difficulties across family members. They do this through aligning observations drawn from inspection of the photographs with specific details from the histories of family members.

In the clinic, the search for familial resemblances is pursued explicitly in the construction of a family tree, begun as described earlier at the home assessment. The following extract in which Lee is discussed illustrates how the family tree can be used:

DR SMITH (CG): [He looks at photographs of Lee.] I'd wondered about Smith-Magennis. But there's nothing very striking to look at ... he's a bit square-ish in the face.

DR LOWE (SPR): Why has it come to light?

DR SMITH: [Examines Lee's family tree.] The mother's sister's son has learning difficulties, maybe I should see him?

Dr Smith states he can see nothing very striking when looking at Lee's photographs. However, after examining the family tree, he juxtaposes information from this source (that the mother's sister's son has learning difficulties) with the fact that Lee's face is 'a bit square-ish'.

This alignment of evidence of a particular facial 'look' with a familial trace of a related problem is enough to strengthen the case for keeping Lee within the genetics clinic, even though his features do not look 'very striking'. Dr Smith draws on the family tree to imply that he can see something in the family that might mean that Lee's problems are inherited. Thus, the idea that features suggestive of a genetic syndrome may be expressed across family members is also incorporated into the family tree.

Conclusions: the dysmorphological gaze

In this chapter I have examined the organization of clinical work and explored how the gaze of dysmorphology is performed in the clinic. What is enacted by the specific processes and practices that we have seen is how dysmorphology is a site in which the 'book of nature' is being read, and 'what is' is being revealed as modes of differentiating the pathological. This helps in the reassociation of the clinic in genetic medicine with the scientific epistemological–ontological relation.

Following Strathern (2009, p.153), we can see much of this work as a 'wonderful rendition of the ontology of perspectivalism'. This is

> *the* Euro-American scientific view that holds that the physical world is continuous, and co-terminous with the universe, the same for everyone, the only shortfall being in knowledge of it, such that diverse experiences are taken as a matter of diverse perspectives on it.

(p.153)

This said, I have shown how deciding upon the appropriate description and classification of individual cases does not entail a straightforward application of a predefined set of clinical parameters. To the contrary, clinical work – and especially the recognition of a syndrome – emerges as rooted in an immersion in the fleshy and material world of the family. In this world of the clinic, doctors and nurses attach to the family – from the home visit, to consultations in the clinic, and discussion at team meetings. Doctors know they must first 'pass' with the family and then, in turn, the family becomes participant in the work of constructing a clinical picture of both the child and itself

When it comes to making sense of the materials assembled through these various aspects of clinical work, I have illustrated how the team juxtaposes and aligns evidence, including patients' features, and draws together details, not just from looking at a patient, but also from constructing a patient's history, examining photographs of the patient and their family, by making a family tree, and by considering the histories of the individuals within the family as well as offering observations of family members. We have also seen how team members examine and debate the clinical details, including photographs of individuals and representations of family trees, and try to establish whether or not what they are seeing is dysmorphia, and whether it is familial. A number of clinic-based technologies are implicated in this work.

The clinical world I portray here is a different world from the clinic performed in the 'fronts' of academic meetings and papers described earlier in Chapter 4. Contrastingly, this is a clinic that does not abstract the doctor or the patient and their families as 'social beings' (Foucault 2003b). Instead what we see is how the clinic is socially immersed and entangled in what Haraway (2007) calls the ordinary and the material. Rather than medicine being transformed into techno-medicine, or reduced to a singular perspective, molecular or otherwise, something goes on in the clinic, when it comes to the diagnosis of dysmorphology at least, which allows multiple perspectives and possibilities to be enacted and to rub up against one another.

This includes both positive and non-positive knowledge. In the clinic doctors engage quite openly in different modes of thought – including subjective assessment – and openly express uncertainty, doubt and contradiction. Rather than maintain a monolithic rationale that attempts to reduce, stabilize and singularize disease processes to one reality, the clinic emerges as a site where multiple methods (not just scientific ones) are enacted.

Critically, what we also see is deferral to clinical perception and judgement, grounded in the material world of the body and the family. Additionally, perception and judgement are collectively produced, not simply embodied by a singular figure. At one moment, the gaze of dysmorphology is enacted as embodied in one physician, just as a syndrome may be seen as embodied by an individual child. In the next, the gaze is distributed across occasions and people, just as the syndrome is distributed across the bodies of the family.

In the face of all this it seems, then, that many commentators completely underestimate the nature of the clinic in genetic medicine. Laboratory and other technologies, such as blood tests, scans or x-rays, certainly give perspectives into the living body, but they require 'reading' to make their relevance explicit: the laboratory may help activate moments where these calculations happen, but it is in the clinic that we see moments of decision and indecision take place.

As outlined in Chapter 2, what is being performed here revives the clinic as a *centre of discretion*. Although the contemporary object of the clinical gaze may, increasingly, focus on the relationships between the observed body and the dispersed images of pathology, we have seen how establishing this relation is enacted as relying upon processes of collective reasoning and adjudication rather than the simple application of prescriptive schemata (see also Atkinson 1995).

7   Rebirthing the clinic

'I loved the cross-harmonies between nature and data. You taught me this. The way signals from a pulsar in deepest space follow classical number sequences, which in turn can describe the fluctuations of a given stock or currency. You showed me this. How market cycles can be interchangeable with the time cycles of grasshopper breeding, wheat harvesting. You made this form of analysis horribly and sadistically precise. But you forgot something along the way.'

'What?'

'The importance of the lopsided, the thing that's skewed a little. You were looking for balance, beautiful balance, equal parts, equal sides. I know this. I know you know. But you should have been tracking the yen in its tics and quirks. The little quirk. The misshape.'

(DeLillo 2003, p.200. Reprinted with the permission of Scribner, a Division of Simon & Schuster, Inc. from COSMOPOLIS by Don DeLillo. Copyright © 2003 by Don DeLillo. All rights reserved.)

Introduction

In Don DeLillo's terms, we have already seen how the clinic in dysmorphology attends to the lopsided, to that which is skewed a little; and how it pays attention to the tics and quirks of bodies, minds and genes.

In this chapter I suggest that in dysmorphology we are witnessing the 'rebirth' of the clinic as a site for the production of knowledge about genetics. The dysmorphology clinic emerges in my analysis as a site in which some of the work of clinical classification is still observable. My observations propose that much of this classificatory work is 'messy', prior to its sedimentation in the 'pure space' of classificatory systems (Bowker and Star 2000), or indeed, even in the calculative space of bioinformatics.

It is important to examine what this 'mess' of classificatory work signifies. It has been suggested that the work of molecular biology would progressively erode the function of clinical judgement and perception in this process of diagnosis and classification. However, as we have already begun to see, the relationship between the laboratory and the clinic appears to be much more mutually co-constituting than is generally recognized. Like the links between the genotype and the phenotype, the relationship between the clinic and the laboratory is in dysmorphology, is far from unilinear or settled. This raises questions about what is accomplished in the way dysmorphology performs the relationship between the clinic and laboratory.

Analysis is particularly important at this point because many studies on genetic medicine focus on the impact of a genetic diagnosis, but do not particularly attend to how, and at what moments, a genetic diagnosis is accomplished. Nor indeed, and just as importantly, do these studies note when it is not accomplished.

In the current case of dysmorphology – against any notion that diagnostics in genetics is a straightforward matter – classification emerges as far from settled. Furthermore, as we have seen in the previous chapter, the performance of clinical expertise in dysmorphology is accompanied by moments of explicit uncertainty, ambiguity and deferral over the identification of the pathological and the attribution of a clinical diagnosis (cf. Bharadwaj 2002; Hedgecoe 2003; Sarangi and Clarke 2002). Indeed, in Don DeLillo's terms (cited above), we have already seen how the clinic in dysmorphology attends to the lopsided, to that which is skewed a little; and how it pays attention to the tics and quirks of bodies, minds and genes.

We can see this attention and care in how families and children are rarely reduced to data. We can also see it in how, in this clinical domain, members do not simply discharge the patient who fails to fit into a specific category. On the contrary, clinicians go to great lengths to legitimate 'keeping patients on'. To do this, as we will see in the rest of this chapter, they have to construct a case for the genetic basis of a patient's features or problems, even if that basis cannot yet be 'proven' or made visible at a molecular or cytogenetic level. Indeed, I am arguing that it is the very complexity of the genetic domain that affords medicine a site in which more medical discretion, not less, is necessary. This is exactly *because* this is a science of the complex and heterogeneous; a medicine whose very focus is on the lopsided, quirky and incomplete.

I should be clear here: I am not identifying the uncertainty and deferral, which are characteristics of clinical process in dysmorphology, as a case study of the failure of science and technology on the ground. On the contrary, I see the analysis as offering an alternative way to understand the significance of explicit ambivalence, uncertainty and deferral over genetic diagnosis. As I am about to show, the clinic is not only equipped to handle uncertainty, but it emerges as a space that actually thrives on the imprecise.

Keeping people on

Diagnostic decisions do not hold because they are true; they are true because they 'hold' (Latour 1989). To hold, they must stand up to normal protocols in the specific science, and they must withstand the critical judgement of the experts in the field. However, the observations of the dysmorphology clinic presented in the previous chapter suggest that deferral is equally important to making a diagnostic decision.

To give an example of this work of deferral, the clinical team in the following extract is sitting together at one of their weekly meetings in the department of medical genetics. They are discussing a young boy, Simon, a 'follow-up':

CARLY (GSN): A follow-up. He's a dysmorphic chap we've looked at together, he's not Smith-Magennis ... He's obese with ADHD [attention deficit hyper-activity disorder] and difficult behaviour, no significant dysmorphic features, I thought about seeing him in a year.

DR SMITH (CG):   How old?

CARLY: Eight.

DR SPRADLEY (SPR):   [Looking at photographs] He's big.

DR SMITH: I remember his photos, leave it more than one, maybe two years. I wouldn't discharge him. He's got a lot of problems, it's worth keeping people on.

The key aspect of this extract that I want to emphasize is the idea of 'keeping people on'. In the absence of a diagnosis, the clinicians are still working to categorize Simon: he is dysmorphic and has many associated problems. The paradox is noteworthy: at the same time as he is 'a dysmorphic chap', he has 'no significant dysmorphic features'.

This paradox relates back to the claim made by dysmorphologists that they are able to see dysmorphia, even where the specifics of a person's features do not fit with the signs of a particular syndrome, as I discussed earlier. Simon has been seen before, he is a 'follow-up'. Although the consultant cannot identify a specific dysmorphic feature, or immediately categorize his problems within a specific syndrome, he still wants to keep Simon on in the clinic and see him in a year's time. He thus identifies him as 'dysmorphic', despite the lack of specific diagnostic characteristics.

Legitimation for this type of manoeuvre may vary. Earlier, in the case of Charles, we saw how he was kept on because Dr Little said he could see some-thing, even though he could not yet verbalize it. On other occasions deferral is justified because the patient is a baby, and they may need to 'grow into the face of a syndrome'. This is because some signs emerge only as the child gets older. In this, the clinic is enacting one of the basic theoretical tropes of developmental biology.

The puzzle in the present case is that Simon is already eight years old and he still does not fit any recognized syndrome; and yet he is being 'kept on'. In this case, it is the clinicians' recognition that the diagnostic categories are in flux that is being performed. Therefore, Simon is being kept on because the knowledge, rather than the child, may change.

Despite there being already over 3,000 named syndromes in the database, dysmorphological categorization is still in its early childhood. Clinical diagnostic categorizations, and the classification of syndromes are still, like babies and chil-dren, 'becomings' (Lee 1998): they are entities *in the making*.

Confirming the genetic

I now turn to exploring the various ways in which deferral and decision are accomplished. This is important, because it is through unpicking these kinds of moves and accounts that we can discover what the dysmorphology clinic is accomplishing, both in relation to its performance of clinical medicine, and in its relation to science.

Keeping a patient on in the clinic in the absence of a firm diagnosis can be achieved by establishing that they are dysmorphic. Diagnostic tests, even when they are available, do not necessarily provide answers that can be treated as unequivocal. First, definitive tests are only available for a limited range of syndromes, so they cannot be used to adjudicate in many cases; and even when such tests do exist, and are used, they are not always treated as definitive. Instead they may be treated as *confirmative*, as in the case of chromosome analysis.

In the extract that follows, for example, the consultant is in the clinic with Mandy, a woman in her thirties who has had surgery on a hole in her heart, her cleft palate, and her vocal chords, and who lives in a care home. Prior to Mandy's arrival, Dr White describes her to the team as 'a query 22Q deletion', pointing out 'she's got the face' and 'the full house' of Di George syndrome.

After a taking her own history and doing a physical examination, the consultant gives Mandy her diagnosis, Velo-Cardio-Facial syndrome[1] (the alternative name for Di George), and that she wants to do some tests. She explains why:

DR WHITE (CG): I don't know if anyone has mentioned any names yet Mandy. The function of the back of your throat is associated with Velo-Cardio-Facial syndrome. This condition is associated with this feature and also very often people with this have heart problems, which you've had. A hole in the heart is typical. People with this condition often have problems at school and also have a tendency to get a little bit depressed ... It is caused by just a little bit of genetic material being missing. So the test is to confirm that you have this small genetic change. [The nurse, Lottie, goes to get pictures of the chromosomes to show Mandy.] *The test is just to confirm we have the diagnosis, there won't be any new surprises.* [Lottie comes back with the folder full of glossy diagramatic pictures of chromosomes, and Dr White uses it to show Mandy a picture of chromosomes and where they reside in the cell.] Basically there is a little piece missing! We all have changes but sometimes we know about it and sometimes we don't. Is there anything you want to ask? Is it making you anxious?

Dr White explains that the symptoms that Mandy displays (hole in the heart, problems with her throat, difficulties at school) fit with a diagnosis of Velo-Cardio-Facial syndrome. She tells Mandy that it is caused by 'just a little bit of genetic material being missing', and that the test she wants to do is to confirm that Mandy has this small genetic change. She says that everyone has changes but they don't notice them. In her account she stresses that the test is confirmatory and that there 'won't be any surprises'. In this instance, then, Dr White enacts the test as confirmative of the clinical picture and her diagnosis, but not as helping her to make the diagnosis.

Keeping the genetic open

At other times, the clinical team may confirm the clinical picture by drawing on evidence to cast doubt on either the relevance or the reliability of a test result. For example, the relevance may be undermined by the strength of a clinical picture. In this instance, rather than rejecting the diagnosis and disposing of the patient, the diagnosis may remain provisional.

Indeed, the clinical team can be seen to move between their readings of the physical features and interpretations of tests in ways that may well privilege 'the clinical picture' rather than the laboratory-based test result. In the following extract, Dr White is doing a consultation with Peter, a 22-year-old man. Peter is a rarity in the clinic because he is an adult. Peter was originally referred to the genetic clinic with a query over whether he has Marfan syndrome,[2] and in the previous consultation Dr White took some blood tests.

DR WHITE: Right. The first time we saw you there was a question you could have Marfan syndrome, but it doesn't look like it. We did some blood tests and looked at your chromosomes and they have come back normal.

PETER: Marvellous.

DR WHITE: And we were looking for Fragile X, sometimes boys can be very tall with that condition, this was normal, so all the tests we have done are normal.

PETER: Marvellous.

In the opening exchange Dr White is giving the results of the tests and of her original diagnostic analysis: Peter does not have Marfan syndrome or Fragile X, the chromosome tests came back as normal which confirms the clinical picture – 'it doesn't look like it [Marfan syndrome]'. Peter doesn't look like Marfan.

Peter says that it is 'marvellous' that the genetic test results are normal. But then the interaction goes on:

DR WHITE: The one concern you had last time was the test you had on your heart, are you still worried?

PETER: No, we're getting through that, they want another scan for the heart.

DR WHITE: That's useful to know, if you weren't [already booked for a heart scan] I might have sent you for another one.[3]

Dr White moves on to Peter's clinical problems with his heart and says that if he wasn't having another scan she would have ordered one herself, thus suggesting that she is not giving him up. Even though the genetic tests were normal Dr White moves the interaction on in a way that opens the case back up:

PETER: Yes, because I had a blackout.

DR WHITE: Tell me about the blackout.

PETER: I don't know much, I was feeding the cat and that's me fell flat [goes on to say that he thinks he was out for about 10 minutes].

DR WHITE: Did they measure your blood pressure?

PETER: Yes, fine, he's put me down for a brain scan because my balance is gone.

DR WHITE: I'm just looking at the notes [looks through a large stack of hospital records].

PETER: The Infirmary [the referring hospital] was supposed to send a letter for me to have my knee done. They can't find it anywhere.

DR WHITE: Let me jot down what is going on.

PETER: [He lists the various problems and investigations out loud and Dr White writes them down in her notes.] Cardiology – ECG; Eyes – OK; MRI of the spine – [Dr White reads out the report and states out loud that '2 discs are bulging']; Referred for physio; Neurological – MRI on brain. [Dr White then looks through the notes for information about his need for a knee operation.]

DR WHITE: We're wondering why you have all these problems. Most of your problems are with your back – we need to look at the MRI [scan]. I think we've done all we can from a genetic point of view. As you say you are very young for disc problems, though you are very tall. I think we'll see you in a year's time to see if the investigations show that there's a particular pattern. We should wait until we have the MRI and repeat heart scan [...] Did we see pictures of when you were younger [to Susan, the GSN]?

SUSAN: Probably.

DR WHITE: I think we should wait for your results.

[Peter leaves, and Dr White tells the nurse and the registrar that 'she's thinking of Sotos'.]

In this phase of the interaction, Dr White gets Peter to report on his recent problems. In this there is a shift from her reporting to him, to him telling her. She then makes a list of these problems and the outstanding investigations that he mentions. Then she switches back to her position as expert, to recover them as possibly of significance to the genetics clinic: 'we are wondering why you have all these problems'. She then tells him she wants to see him in a year's time with all his new scans, even though 'we have done all we can from the genetic point of view'.

When he leaves the clinic, however, she says to the others that she thinks it is Sotos. Since she does not convey this information to Simon, we can presume that this possibility is being entertained more in terms of a deferral than a decision.

Sotos syndrome is also called cerebral gigantism and is a rare genetic disorder caused by mutation in a gene on chromosome 5. It is characterized by excessive physical growth during the first few years of life. Thus chromosomal tests would not show it up – the mutation is too small. And it is a mutation, rather than a bit missing or a bit extra. Dr White wants to check pictures of Peter when he was a child – the implication is that this is because children with Sotos syndrome tend to be large at birth and are often taller, heavier, and have larger heads (macrocrania) than is normal for their age (see Figure 6.2, page 96). This is more difficult to 'see' in a fully grown adult. There is no definitive genetic test for Sotos, which is possibly why she comments that, 'we have done all we can from the genetic point of view'. But Dr White keeps Peter's case open through getting him to bring all his clinical problems back into play, together with the fact he is tall, and alongside the need to wait for the results of the other clinical investigations. Through these moves in which she enrols Peter in the definition of clinical problems, she constructs a formal process of deferral through which she is able to keep him on in the clinic.

Setting aside test results

Sometimes clinicians also cast doubt on a test result. Casting doubt on a test can occur in a number of ways. For example, at another team meeting, a consultant and a specialist nurse discuss the case of a family who may have a genetic syndrome known as Fragile X. It emerged from their discussion that the results from the laboratory test were unclear because they (the laboratory) 'couldn't do a Southern blot'. However, the distinguishing features of Fragile X could be traced in the family, for example, the specialist nurse reports from her home visit and the family history that the mother 'appears to have some learning difficulties' and that 'there are affected nieces and nephews'.

In this case, although the genetic test results were unclear, other materials were brought in to support a diagnosis of Fragile X. Specifically, information in the family tree and observations from the home visit indicate that the family may have the genetic syndrome, which reinforces the provisional diagnosis. In this way, a negative test result does not rule out a provisional clinical diagnosis where other evidence can be brought into consideration, such as family history. Thus the team assemble the evidence in ways which suggest that what is being represented is an aberrant genetic sequence, even if the particular sequence has not yet been mapped, and cannot yet be 'seen' using molecular or cytogenic testing.

Similarly, in the case of Alan, the laboratory test is negative but the clinical picture is strongly indicative:

DR SMITH (CG): Myotonic dystrophy [caused by one of two types of inherited genetic mutations]. Grip problems, cataracts, frontal balding.
PENNY (GSN): The full house almost but the bloods were negative.

Here the consultant aligns the clinical evidence (grip problems, cataracts and frontal balding) to support the diagnosis of myotonic dystrophy. Alan almost has the 'full house', even though the 'bloods were negative': the implication of this is that molecular analysis was unable to detect one of the two genetic changes associated with the diagnosis. However, the team believe it is there – they can 'see' the evidence of a syndrome in the patient.

A negative laboratory test result can sometimes lead to discharge, but is not enough in itself: it has to be associated with other evidence. For example, in the case of Lindsay:

PENNY (GSN): [She describes a child who has mild dysmorphic features.] But he looks OK on these. [She hands round two family photographs to the rest of the team.]

DR GATES (CG): There's nothing, Fragile X and chromosomes have been done, the results are OK.

DR YOUNG (SPR): [Looking at photographs] Ooh! [indicating she finds the baby attractive]

DR GATES: He's not very dysmorphic.

PENNY: [She agrees and adds] The child's father had retinitis pigmentosa 6 years ago. I checked with the mother if the child had any problems, but she's got enough on her plate.

The clinical team does not see the child's features as being dysmorphic and these observations confirm the negative test results, which like the photographs are also 'OK'. This information is also interpreted in the context of the family; the nurse suggests that it may not be appropriate to pursue a diagnosis because the child's mother has 'enough on her plate'. In response, the team moves away from a genetic diagnosis and Lindsay is discharged from the clinic.

The analysis to date indicates that where a patient does not fit neatly into a clinical category, this does not mean that they are to be fully discharged from the clinic. On the contrary, the clinical picture can be assembled in ways that legitimate deferral, so that a patient is 'kept on'. I have also illustrated how the molecular evidence itself is not necessarily relied upon: where there is negative molecular evidence, but the clinical picture of a possible genetic disorder is thought to be strong, a diagnosis is not excluded, but will remain provisional.

Stabilizing diagnosis

It has emerged that, in the field of dysmorphology, it is often difficult to give a definitive genetic diagnosis. As I have shown, where laboratory tests of any kind are used, they are not privileged in any way as definitive forms of evidence. Rather, we have seen how the clinical team moves between different forms of evidence in their assessment of any particular case.

Critically, the significance of any particular aspect of the evidence of dysmorphism has to be established through aligning it within a wider array of clinical data. It appears that the judgement and skill of the clinical team in making a case for the clinical picture is privileged over any single technology.

These complexities are amplified by something about genetic categorization itself. While a tentative, working diagnosis is usually dependent upon the recognition of a pattern of abnormalities, a large number of syndromes share many abnormalities. In addition, there may also be a wide variability in how an abnormality is expressed across different individuals with the same syndrome. The shared nature of many abnormalities, such as learning disability, together with the huge variation in the clinical picture, creates both opportunities and constraints on the clinical team. This complexity can increase the need for judgement and perception. For example:

DR JONES (CG): I've done some research on these three [he points to a pile of files for three children with dysmorphic features], there are 40 possibles [diagnostic categories] for this one, 50 for the other and 38 for that. [He has fed their patterns of abnormalities into a dysmorphology database.]

This indicates that the possibilities are vast. Indeed, overlap between syndromes as well as variation across phenotypes only intensifies the need for clinical judgement. For example, in the following extract the clinical team once again discuss the young boy, Lee:

DR SMITH (CG): [He gets out two photographs from the file, examines them and passes them to the SpR.]
CARLY (GSN): In the photograph I couldn't take from the family [at the home visit] he looks different.
DR SMITH: Thin upper lip.
CARLY: We've seen part of the family before, the father had RP [retinitis pigmentosa].
DR PALLING (SPR): Are you thinking more Smith-Magennis than Prader-Willi?
DR SMITH: More Smith-Magennis
DR PALLING: No, but not very Smith-Magennis either.
DR SMITH: These phenotypes are getting more elastic.

Thus, Lee remains on the perimeter of two different syndromes, because, as the consultant notes, to fix the configuration of abnormalities within one syndrome is difficult, these classifications are subject to change: 'these phenotypes are getting more elastic'.

This ambiguity creates the opportunity for Lee to be held within the genetic ground. Further opportunity for deferral is created by overlap and variation; where the clinical picture does not fit one syndrome, another can be tried. For example, Kyle has been considered for a number of diagnoses since referral to the team:

DR WHITE (CG): Someone who I think has Costello's. Originally he was query Noonan's, he does have some Noonan's features, Costello's is similar. [Adds that he had shown the photographs to two colleagues but they were non-committal.]
PENNY (GSN): The child has major feeding problems.
DR WHITE: I'll tout them [the photos] round again.

No diagnosis had been confirmed for Kyle, although Noonan's had been suspected. However, Costello's is 'similar' to Noonan's and the child may also fit this classification. Furthermore, the discovery of 'major feeding problems' renews the team's interest and this may be the additional information the team need to firm up a diagnosis, because major feeding problems can signify neuro-developmental behavioural problems.

These moments of ambiguity and undecideability create a space of deferral that legitimates the need for more expertise and more technology through which to differentiate the genetic and so fix genetic diagnoses. The consultant decides to keep Kyle on and 'tout the photographs around again' at meetings with other experts.

The clinical laboratory?

I now want to discuss how my analysis of the clinic in genetic medicine suggests that it is being reborn as a site for the production and disposal of knowledge, not for just its consumption. These findings should not surprise.

As discussed in Chapter 2, Foucault (2003a) suggests that the clinic was born as the location of scientific medicine and the discovery of positive knowledge about the body and pathology. In his analysis the clinic is the site of production, producing both medical scientific method and medical knowledge.

However, my findings conflict sharply with much current thinking, in which the relationship between the clinic and science is increasingly being (re)presented in a similar way to the relation between the farm and the laboratory in Latour's (1988) study of the pasteurization of France – as 'remote control' (Cooper 1992). Within this view, the work of the clinic is no longer involved in the production of medical knowledge. Diagnosis has been made remote, and this perspective on the contemporary clinic has been expressed by Armstrong (2007), but is most stridently echoed by Rose:

> 'Medicine' itself has also been transformed. It has become technomedicine, *highly dependent* on sophisticated diagnostic and therapeutic equipment. It has been *fractured* by a complex division of labour among specialists. Doctors have *lost* the monopoly of the diagnostic gaze and of the therapeutic calculation: the clinical judgment of the practicing physician is *hemmed in* and *constrained* by the demands of evidence-based medicine and the requirements for the use of standardized, corporately framed diagnostic and prescribing procedures.
>
> (2007b, pp.10–11, emphases added)

For Rose, medicine is not simply being transformed, but is actually presented as losing its power: it is 'fractured', 'lost', 'hemmed in', 'constrained', 'colonized', 'reshaped'.

Rose writes categorically – as though the effects he asserts are totalizing. In a two-page summary of the state of medicine in the 21st century, he asserts that the 'golden age' of the medical gaze and discretion is long gone. As mentioned in Chapter 3, he suggests 'the treatment of health and illness' has become 'merely another field for calculations of corporate profitability'. He sees capitalization, technologization, and the profound molecularization of 'styles of biomedical thought, judgment and intervention' as executing the takeover of medicine.

What we have seen in dysmorphology is something far more complex: clearly not all doctors have 'lost' the monopoly of the diagnostic gaze and of the thera-peutic calculation. Nor is there evidence in my study of the clinical judgement of practicing physicians being 'hemmed in' and 'constrained' by the demands of evidence-based medicine and the requirements for the use of standardized, corpo-rately framed diagnostic and prescribing procedures. In the place of contempo-rary forms of medical disposal and decision-making, in which the display of expertise entails speedy closure. In the genetic clinic I have found instead a slow-ing down of clinical process, and explicit moments of undecidability, uncertainty and instability over genetic diagnostic categories.

At the same time as there is a commitment to the possibility of certainty, of fixing diagnostic categories in grids and codes through the future development of technoscience, clinical practice within dysmorphology is performing something about the genetic clinic that is highly significant and related as much to its modes of deferral as to its forms of decision. This is to suggest, tentatively and provi-sionally, how undecidability, uncertainty and instability of genetic diagnosis are a prominent feature of dysmorphology.

This deliberate sustaining of ambiguity and uncertainty within the clinic requires additional explanation, especially when it appears to run alongside a firm commitment to a future of diagnostic certainty. In my view, it is precisely these moments of ambiguity and uncertainty that help to hold patients on the 'genetic ground' and establish the very space of deferral which is needed to secure that future. A future in which classification becomes sedimented in a technoscience that will continue to press back the boundaries of the genomic unknown, but a technoscience which also creates opportunities for more clinical judgement to secure its proper interpretation and salience.

Members in the clinic create a space of deferral in which the genetic itself is performed as very much still open, and its categories as revisable. Thus, the dysmorphology clinic emerges as a site in which we can observe the complex, practical work of classification. Clinical uncertainty and the trope of deferral mean that the logic of the clinic appears to call for advances in technoscience that foreshadow its own demise. This is the way of the clinic. It performs an apparent commitment to future facts, which will be secured in the laboratory that is yet to come.

Critically, this projection is itself always being deferred. This deferral creates the space in which the clinic and pathological entities are irreducible to molecular biology. I am showing this in complete contrast to commentators, such as Rose who presses how medicine is *being reconfigured by a profound 'moleculariza-tion' of styles of biomedical thought, judgment, and intervention* (Rose 2007, p.11, emphasis added).

For the moment the boot is on the other foot. Rather than deferring to the laboratory, it is the laboratory that must travel to the clinic, in order to be noted, interpreted, or even discarded. It is the laboratory that is behind and slow to catch up to the complexity of what is being seen in the clinic. Not the other way around.

Conclusion

In this chapter I have shown how dysmorphology clinical work does not merely fit patients into extant diagnostic categories. This finding is important because it has prompted me to reconsider how the dysmorphology clinic performs the relationship between science, technology and clinical work, in a way that is itself of significance.

Specifically, through a focus on how different forms of evidence are produced and brought into play in the dysmorphology clinic, I have shown how clinical work involves identifying and naming which patterns of physical features and other effects may have a genetic origin, and which do not. Further, drawing on typical cases, I have explored how patients are held on the genetic ground even in the absence of a definitive diagnosis. Indeed, in the cases where it is available, it is possible that molecular or chromosomal evidence be discredited as inadequate. Thus, clinicians perform the technoscience of the laboratory as, at times, creating the need for more moments of interpretation, and more moments of clinical discretion, rather than less.

At the same time as genetic clinical process is performed in ways that privilege clinical perception over other kinds of technology, moments of ambiguity and uncertainty over diagnosis create 'a space of deferral'. This space of deferral serves to legitimate a future in which even more technoscience – and consequently more clinical judgement – is called on to differentiate the genetic, and amend or determine genetic diagnoses.

When performed as a new frontier of medical knowledge, the alignment of the gene and the clinic creates a space of interpretation that in turn produces the opportunity for a reinvigoration of clinical power. Thus, the conception of the 'death of the clinic' is premature. The clinic in dysmorphology is being reperformed as a site of knowledge production in the identification and classification of disease entities. Furthermore, as will be seen in the chapter that follows, it is precisely the non-relation between the genotype (the abstraction of informational codes) and the phenotype (the mess of distributed fleshy substance) that affords medicine its place as a site of crossing and translation in the production of the genetic as a new sphere of life.

8   Dysmorphology's portraits

The form in which truth is originally shown is the surface in which relief is both manifested and abolished – the portrait.

(Foucault 2003a, p.5)

Introduction

In this chapter I explore the kinds of bodies and medical entities that process and practice in dysmorphology perform. This continues the analysis of genetic medicine in the last chapter, where initial findings pointed to the clinic acting as a centre of discretion and rebutted the rather superficial prognosis that the clinic was being transformed into an outpost of the laboratory, in which clinical judgement is neither relevant nor necessary.

In what follows I examine the specificity of how the clinic constructs the clinical pictures they make and 'read' as representations of the real. I do this by considering these clinical pictures as a new form of *portraiture*. Shifting to thinking of the clinical pictures that dysmorphologists make as forms of portraiture is important because, as Jordonova suggests (2000, 2003), it emphasizes that they are constructions: 'portraits are always art – that is, they are not natural depictions of a state of affairs in the world but creations' (Jordonova 2003, p.47).

However, we must not treat these portraits as mere simulacra. Rather, by considering them portraits, we can consider clinical pictures as material, mobile, semiotic objects that are produced in a specific cultural and social time-space location. Moreover, examining how these portraits are constructed allows us to examine the culturally and socially specific *ideas* that they make manifest and circulate.

In what follows I illuminate how dysmorphology's portraits are constructed, and consider what it is that they accomplish. Firstly, I show how the portraits put into a play a way of seeing bodies and their parts as the substantive and fleshy manifestations of genes. Secondly, I argue that my analysis of these portraits helps to make visible the way in which the clinic is a site of crossing and translation between the molecular (the genotype) and the molar (the phenotype), between the abstract and the substantial, and between informational codes and flesh. What I suggest these methods of portraiture both reflect and constitute is the shift in genetic science from one gene as responsible for one disease, to the complexity of classifying a syndrome-phenotype as the expression of a genotype. Thus, the portrait in dysmorphology, offers the figure of a syndrome-genotype relation, that is genetic and connected to reproduction, but does not necessarily have the characteristics of Mendelian forms of inheritance. It is a way of representing syndromes as not reducing either to a single gene or to the figure of an individual and, instead, emerges in its partial connection between the assemblage and juxtaposition of materials deriving from different bodies. In this we can see how the clinic is doing the '*new* genetics'.

Texts and surfaces

Ahead of this analysis, I need to say something more about those who see the clinic as abandoning the flesh. In her now notorious (and often misquoted) passage, Haraway (1991) states that it is time to write the 'Death of the Clinic'. She pictures the 'loss' of medical dominance quite differently from the analysis offered by Rose in the previous chapter. As Haraway (1991, p.194) puts it, '[t]he old dominations of white capitalist patriarchy seem nostalgically innocent now' since, in normalizing heterogeneity (e.g., into man and woman, white and black), such dominations at least provided a space of subjectivity, a depth.

Particularly compelling in Haraway's more sophisticated rendering is her vision of the normless world of 'texts and surfaces' to which medical dominance, for all its normalizing effects, is giving way:

> 'Advanced capitalism' and post-modernism release heterogeneity without a norm, and we are flattened, without subjectivity, which requires depth, even unfriendly and drowning depths. It is time to write the Death of the Clinic. The clinic's methods required bodies and works; we have texts and surfaces. Our dominations don't work by medicalization and normalization anymore; they work by networking, communications redesign, stress management.
>
> (Haraway 1991, p.194)

Haraway sees the clinic's death in the emerging shift from biology as clinical practice (requiring bodies and work), to biology as inscription (information sound bites, technobabble, and the embedding and totalizing association of advanced capitalism and postmodernism).

The theory that we are experiencing (and as Haraway implies, should be resisting) an epochal shift from flesh, substance, depth and subjectivity, to the digitalizing of life and an information age is well rehearsed in the literature. Rheinberger (2000) goes so far as to suggest an epochal shift in which the molecularization of biology (and therefore medicine) augurs the demise of the nature/culture divide, so that the natural and the social can no longer be seen as ontologically different:

> What is new about molecular biological writing is that we now gain access to the texture, and hence the calculation, instruction and legislation of the

human individual's organic existence, that is to a script that until now it has been the privilege of evolution to write, to rewrite and to alter.

(p.28)

From this perspective of life being reduced to informational codes, the programming of bodies emerges as *plastic*: the 'real' is no longer the flesh but is the script, or the code. In this way the gene appears as something technological, object-like, unnatural, inorganic – not fleshy at all.

Intervention using the new genetic and reproductive technologies is represented as operating at the level of *instruction*, rather than at the level of the performance of metabolic processes (Rheinberger 1997). The language here shifts too: clinical interventions need to be 'smart' and 'intelligent', able to 'switch' genes on and off; contrastingly, old clinical technologies are figured as blunderbusses.

This is the language of IT – a language that penetrates how people in disciplines like cancer genetics talk to each other and to publics. It is racy and slick. Even, dare one say it, inhuman. This language attaches medicine to the world of the digital machine. Here the basis of life bares no resemblance to Canguilhem's (1991) normativity: there is nothing vital here (see also Greco 2009) and everything is mere abstraction and simulacrum. It belongs to the new fronts of medicine, such as the Gene Knowledge Parks discussed in Chapter 3, far away from the messy work of the clinic, and the flesh and complexity of children and families.

Fleshing up representation

This foregoing representation of science as only molecular forgets that biology is itself clunky, partial, material and incomplete. As we are already learning from the analysis in the previous chapters, however, bioscience is far from being similar to a computer game – if it were scientists would not need to move between animal models, living organisms, the laboratory and the computer. And we would not need systems biology and epigenetics to help us move past the fallacy that mapping the genome would solve all our problems.

Discourses about the molecularization of biology and medicine seem to be underpinned by two presumptions: firstly, that molecular biology has become dominant in ways that obliterate other kinds of bio-knowledge and understandings; and, secondly, that this dominance has dematerialized medicine and turned it away from flesh, bodies and work and towards informational codes, digits and maths. It is as though persons and their bodily troubles can no longer be healed or enhanced as flesh, or even as cyborgs, but only engineered as virtual avatars.

These twin processes do not only strip away the flesh, but are presumed to take the ground from under the feet of medicine. The supposition in all this, as has already been discussed, is that medicine's dominant place in society is under threat. But surely it is more important and interesting to explore how the clinic continues to function and what place it has in the so-called information age? As Chatterji *et al.* (1998) argue: 'how the clinic is maintained as an idea and a practice in day-to-day functioning in different societal contexts ... within which we could see how the new ideologies of domination through information, require and use bodies' (p.171).

As we have been observing in the study of dysmorphology, not all the flesh is stripped away. At least, not all of the time. We have already witnessed how clinical process in genetic medicine continuously shifts, back and forth, between fleshy bodies and different forms of representation of these bodies, their parts, and how they are functioning, including chromosomal and molecular tests. Specifically, many photographs and slides of babies and children, parts of their bodies, and photographs of other family members and parts of their bodies, are juxtaposed with other visual imagery, such as family trees, in the construction of a clinical picture.

Alongside this visual imagery, doctors and others give their accounts and inter-pretations. I have reported in Chapters 6 and 7 how these clinical pictures are being assembled by clinicians as ways of detecting the presence, or absence, of a syndrome. While simulacra are treated in medicine as a part of the real, as Grace (2003) argues, we have seen dysmorphologists enact their readings of the repre-sentations of photographs and scans as though they were representations of the real, not simulacrums. Indeed, as mentioned before, they tend to reject the simu-lacra of new computer technologies in preference of diagnosing syndromes from the faces of people, as if they are like any other natural objects: legible to a scientific and disciplined gaze.

Medicine and portraiture

The dysmorphology clinic constructs a very specific form of portraiture: *assem-blages* in which various kinds of bodies and their parts are juxtaposed in multiple and heterogeneous images. Inasmuch as this form of portraiture differs from earlier forms of medical portraiture, which typically mimic other classical forms of portraiture in showing a singular figure rendered in great and vivid detail, these differences require attention because of what this clinical form of assemblage is bringing into presence.

As the following quotation from Thomas Sydenham indicates, medicine's use of portraits is nothing new:

> 'He who writes the history of diseases must ... observe attentively the clear and natural phenomena of diseases, however uninteresting they may seem. In this he must imitate the painters who when they paint a portrait are careful to mark the smallest signs and natural things that are to be found on the face of the person they are painting'.[1]

> (cited in Foucault 2003a, p.5)

There is a long history of the use of images in clinical work in the science of modelling and visualizing disease and, in calling attention to Sydenham, Foucault is suggesting that the portrait is a powerful technology for circulating knowledge.

Early representations of diseased bodies were either painted or engraved. Like the honorific portraits of individuals, or groups of individuals, which we see hanging in universities, corporation board rooms, stately homes and galleries (Sekula 1986), traditional medical portraits usually portray a figure of an individual. As a well accepted clinical method, through which diseases are constructed and a model fabricated, these portraits would illustrate medical textbooks along with illustrations of a particular affected part.

Sometimes these portraits are classic depictions of a human figure in a specific pose, such as Charcot's famous portrait of hysteria depicting Augustine in ecstasy (see Didi-Huberman 2004). Here the figure performs a particular relation between the appearance of the person and their essence: and the suggestion is that how the figure looks, and how they are as a person, is being determined. They are, perhaps, being 'consumed' by the pathology, or possibly vice versa – the pathology is consuming them. Therefore, the portrait could also suggest that the pathology is an effect of their essence.

Whichever way round, the figure of an individual is taken to stand for a disease and typify some of its signs and symptoms. The whole person personifies the disease, while representations of specific signs exemplify what makes up the disease – its constituent parts. Gilman (1988), however, presses us to attend to the implicit cultural and social significance of how clinical science has deployed portraits of 'affected' persons in the work of *establishing* pathologies. Here the specific use of photographs has had some importance because they have an epistemological significance as depictions of the real, rather than as simulations.

Portraiture and photography

Photography expanded upon these early representational practices by depicting types, characters and pathologies. Photographic representations of organs and lesions, largely used to illustrate textbooks and atlases of pathology, have become standard practice, with trained medical illustrators/photographers forming a part of health care teams.

Importantly, it was the typical case or classic presentation of a pathological condition which was captured even in the earliest years of photographic technology and have been increasingly used ever since. Photography was used to compile extensive typologies of characters and social types. These earlier photographs often depicted an individual figure in a pose: the figure *typified* the presentation of a disease or condition.

Photographs, which appear to capture and reproduce 'the real', help to associate what is displayed with the truth – unmediated, for example, by an artist's art. Because the epistemological status of photographs is hard to dispute (Cohen and Meskin 2004), they help reinforce that an accurate portrayal of a given object is being depicted in the clinic.

The attempt within medicine, particularly physiognomy, to identify and classify pathologies of character and temperament through physical appearance also has a history here. Appearance was thought to reveal the inner character of the person, and, as Kemp and Wallace (2000, p.94) suggest, 'philosophy, science and medicine have been consistently mobilized over the ages to provide a framework of explanation of how inner is expressed in outer'. Here I should also mention phrenology, in which the skull's shape and form was mapped, based on the belief that areas on the skull, together with their size and shape, were indicative of different faculties and character traits. Duster (1990) has likened DNA mapping of criminals, and the population searches for genetic markers of criminal types, to phrenology.

Two well-known early examples of the way in which photographs were used in linking inner pathology to outer appearance are Lombroso (1835–1909) and Galton (1882–1911). Lombroso equated criminality and physiognomic types by codifying variation in human appearance into a classification of types, in which criminal traits were correlated with visible physical indices. Francis Galton combined the resources of photography with anthropometric techniques to classify human types, called 'composite portraits' (http://galton.org/composite.htm). Composite portraiture was a method of analysing the images of different persons identified as belonging to a particular category of person, such as sick or criminal or a leader, so that the ideal type could be ascertained. This face could then be used as a way of recognizing someone as belonging to a particular category or not. For example, if their face did not match the ideal face typifying a leader, their selection for officer rank in the armed forces could be questioned.

Although Lombroso and Galton were interested in the classification of types, and in the correspondence between appearance and character, they were also interested in the hereditary transmission of character from generation to generation. One of Lombroso's methods, for example, was to transform the photographic family album and the family tree into the visual display of physiological and phrenological semiology (Lombroso and Lombroso-Ferrero 1972). Indeed, Galton was especially influential in the application of Darwinian ideas and the promotion of eugenic science (e.g. Galton 1904). So the body–world relation that comes into view is between appearance, character, pathology and hereditary.

The depiction of the insane was also a major site for the photographic recording of the relation between appearance and pathology. Asylum patients were photographed in abundance from the middle of the nineteenth century, notably by Hugh Welch Diamond in England, who was one of the founders of the Royal Photographic Society. In addition, and just as famously, an extensive photographic record supplemented Charcot's displays of living patients at the Salpêtrière. In collaboration with photographers Bourneville, Regnard and Londe, Charcot established a photographic unit at the hospital and the publication of *New Iconography of the Salpêtrière* enshrined a voluminous record of the hysterics, cataleptics and other inmates.[2]

The pathology and the body–person relation performed in these kinds of portraits seems totalizing. Despite this, the relation between appearance and essence is not a straightforward one, as we saw in the previous chapter. The art of the clinical gaze is precisely to be able to distinguish and differentiate between appearance and essence. Just as, for Talcott Parsons (1951), one of the cornerstones of medical dominance and medicine's social contract is to be able to weed out and legitimate the genuinely sick from the non-genuine, the key work in the case of dysmorphology is to differentiate the (possibly) syndromic from the rest.

Reading across images

Predominantly these kinds of portraits individuate: the pathology is performed as being located in some *one*, in a singular figure. In this way the pathology is being portrayed as inherent to the body (and mind) of this particular person. These are medicine's usual portraits – their 'representative subjects'. And we have seen throughout the book examples of these in the different photographs I have included along the way, such as the faces of Coffin-Lowry or Sotos syndromes (Figure 1.1 and Figure 6.2 respectively).

These portraits also settle all the parts – the signs, and the symptoms of the pathology – into a whole, complete and reductive medical entity, for example, 'hysteria'. So much so that the figure is taken not so much to represent themselves, but as representing the medical category to which they are being assigned: the figure of the person is being read as signifying the pathology. Foucault (2003a) captures the radical nature of this shift:

> The first structure provided by classificatory medicine is the flat surface of perpetual simultaneity. *Table and picture ... It is a space in which analogies define essences. The picture resembles things, but they also resemble one another.*
>
> (p.5, emphasis added)

This is the meaning that a medical portrait captures. Meaning does not come from the representation of the person being portrayed, but comes instead from its similarity and difference to other representations. There is not simply a likeness of the patient to portray. There is even the possibility that a pathological condition can be represented, settled and fixed in a moment of time (just as a photographic portrait fixes someone in a moment of time) in order to portray something of their essence. What is important is that the picture resembles other pictures of people with the same diagnosis.

The key point is that the pathology can be recognized *as a pathology* by reference not to the persons being portrayed, but to the grid of other pathologies. Likeness is read *across* pathologies more than it is read from portrait to person. This is why juxtaposition is so important, which I will make central in the following analysis. Dysmorphologists use juxtaposition as a part of making 'assemblages' (Deleuze and Parnet 1987), in which different images are juxtaposed or held apart. They do this to read across images in order to see their syndromes.

Consequently, dysmorphologists use photographs in their work in the clinic in a quite different way to traditional medicine. We have seen in the previous chapters on dysmorphology how processes of diagnosis assemble different and multiple images of people and their parts, including their relations. Some family photographs may have been supplied by the nurse from her home visit, and placed in the notes. Other images derive from the examination of the child during consultations. These assemblages unsettle an idea of a disease process as located in a singular body, an individual. What comes into view is the distributed and unsettled nature of a syndrome, which I will now discuss.

Assemblage and juxtaposition

As I described in Chapter 5 about the construction of a history, a typical dysmorphology examination 'starts from the top'. We also heard from Professor Fox how this may entail making themselves 'human', sitting a child on their lap for example, or making the examination into a game with bangles. Typically, the clinical geneticist carefully inspects the head, the face, the tongue, hands, trunk and back, joints, and feet. Measurements are also taken; clinicians are looking at the shape, size and position of features. After this examination the clinician frequently takes photographs of any distinctive features, and may also ask parents for additional photographs of the child when they were younger, of siblings, and of other family members, where these have not already been supplied.

As is evident in Chapters 5 and 6, diagnoses are developed over time and are discussed at length at clinical meetings: they are almost never offered immediately at a clinical consultation. Diagnostic process includes both the assemblage of images together with other clinical materials, such as scans of organs and bones, blood and cytogenic tests, and medical family trees or pedigrees. Different materials are thus juxtaposed so that they can be considered in relation to one another.

Juxtapositions may include either images with images, or images and other materials including laboratory tests. Typically the purpose appears to be to illuminate incongruity and ambiguity as much as it is to elicit conformity. For example, in Chapter 6 it became evident that juxtaposition may be made in ways that either confirm or falsify evidence, such as tests, or a previous diagnosis. These processes of assemblage and juxtaposition can be seen across local clinical meetings, in clinical databases, and in poster and oral presentations at national and international conferences.

At these moments of assemblage (whether in clinical meetings or at academic occasions), clinicians may designate certain forms and shapes as abnormal or unusual. Shapes of interest include the distribution of bodily features (faces, hearts, hands, feet, hair, genitals, brains, skin). Sometimes clinicians, as noted already, typify a child as an 'FLK' – a 'funny looking kid' – or as 'looking a bit chromosomal'. In these assemblages, clinicians are associating features together to see if there is a pattern – a pattern that corresponds to the defining features of a syndrome, one that is known or not yet fully known. Sometimes, as in the cases of Fiona (p.97) and Anna (p.98), the child and their family may simply look syndromic.

Establishing whether the features displayed can be taken to represent a syndrome is a complex process. The pattern-making associates different parts of bodies with each other across systems, such as specific shapes of eyes with abnormalities in brain shapes, and so on and so forth. Many syndromes involve developmental problems: flesh develops in abnormal ways to produce abnormalities in the shapes of organs, such as the brain, and other fleshy parts. It is these abnormal shapes that produce abnormalities in what the clinicians designate as the development of the child (physical, behavioural, intellectual).

Differentiating the cause of abnormality includes establishing whether the 'look' of someone, or one part of them, is also 'in the family'. Here clinicians are looking to see if the sign of a syndrome or a distinguishing feature of an individual are manifest in other family members. Dysmorphologists compare looks and features across family members and then hold them against databases of syndromes.

Clinicians draw upon these clinical methods of assemblage to differentiate when what is abnormal or unusual about bodies, parts, persons and even families, represents a phenotype. This is because, for the most part, as already discussed, there is no genetic technology (molecular test) that can make anomalies visible at the molecular level (see also Reardon and Donnai 2007). Through the enactment of rational detachment, geneticists make patterns out of the way a person and/or the members of their family look. They are looking for signs that represent the defining features of a syndrome.

I want to suggest that a relation between the particular features of a syndrome, the notion of a phenotype (as the expression of an atypical, aberrant genotype) is fabricated in the mode of juxtaposition rather than that merely of comparison. To recap, a phenotype for geneticists is the way that a genotype is manifested: it is the substantial or fleshy expression of a genotype, a specific arrangement of protein expressed as codes and numbers. Therefore indicators such as low IQ, a big head or the distribution of hair may be read less as an individual feature, and more as a sign, and evidence, of a syndrome in the family.

If a particular feature is read as part of a pattern of features, and thus is judged to be evidence of a syndrome, the question arises as to whether it is genetic. And then, of course, whether – if it is genetic – it is inherited. If it is inherited, then there is the issue of 'morphological risk' (Löwy 1996) and the question of whether or not the aberration can be passed on down the generations and through a family line.

In summary, what is implicated by how geneticists assemble their clinical pictures is that how people look and how their bodies function (the phenotype) may not just be evidence of a syndrome. What is also being suggested by how these assemblages juxtapose particular signs is that the syndrome may be the effect of a specific aberrant (but as yet invisible) genotype, a syndrome–genotype relation.

Investigating the syndrome–genotype relation

It is this relation, the syndrome–genotype, which dysmorphology's portraits evoke. They do this at moments through the way in which assemblages juxtapose particular representations of bodies and their parts, even where there is no definitive evidence of such a relation (such as a cytogenetic or molecular test).

The aberrations that are being suggested by these juxtapositions may be as tiny as a single gene defect, or 'huge' where, to use the locution of one expert, 'a bit of chromosome has fallen off and landed in the wrong place'.[3]

The following extract helps to illustrate how portraiting the possibility of a syndrome–genotype relation is being discussed at a local clinical meeting. In this meeting people from across the service and the different clinics come together to present their cases to each other, and look at 'slides' (the images collected from the different cases that each team is involved in). Dr Little and Dr Smith (consultant geneticists), Dr Grey and Dr Milne (specialist registrars in genetics) are present. Like Dysmorphology Club, discussion and debate over interpretations and diagnoses are the norm at these meetings. In the following extracts the team are discussing Poppy:

[Dr Grey sets up the projector. They go through a number of new referrals as well as ongoing cases. Dr Grey moves the slides on to show a picture of an 8-year-old girl, Poppy, with short brown hair grinning into the camera. This is the case Dr Little is very excited about.]

DR SMITH: Would anyone like to make a diagnosis?

DR LITTLE: This is Poppy, she is doing very well, she's in a regular class, she has some help but is not coping. She came with her mum and dad who want to know what's wrong. Poppy was referred by a number of doctors and by a community health worker who suggested I should see her and mentioned that there was something odd about Mum too.

[Dr Little projects a slide of a head shot of Poppy, then a slide of her hands, palms down.]

DR GREY: Short finger.

DR LITTLE: A short finger, how about the nail? … [no comment from the others] it's more deeply embedded than the others.

[Slide of Poppy's hands, palm facing up.]

DR MILNE: Foetal finger pads…

DR LITTLE: Short thumbs.

[Slide of left foot.]

DR LITTLE: Short toes and broad.

DR MILNE: Shapeless feet.

DR LITTLE: Tiny, smaller than her younger sister … also the toenails are deeply embedded, the parents commented on how difficult it was to cut them.

Up to this point the team have been looking at slides of Poppy. These assemble images of her face, her profile, her hands and fingers, and her feet. Although asked to make a diagnosis, no one proffers a suggestion. Then the slide show moves on:

[Slide of the child's mother – head shot of woman in her 30s with short curly hair and large eyes framed by large glasses – the doctors all exclaim when they see this slide.]

DR LITTLE: She has large eyes, lateral aversion of the eyes [she demonstrates by pulling her own eyes to the side to illustrate an oriental look], her height is 1.49 [metres]. I got hold of the mother's baby notes, she was seen by lots of paediatricians because of her short stature and her pictures were shown at national dysmorphology meetings in the 70s. So that's Mum.

[Side profile of the mother – Dr Little comments on her prominent eyebrows that have high and large arches.]

DR SMITH: We're talking about Kabuki aren't we, but the nose isn't.

DR LITTLE: The girl [Poppy] does [have the nose] ... I'm encouraging Mum to get some pictures of her[self] as a child.

The moment that Dr Little puts up a slide of Poppy's mother the rest of the team exclaim. As mentioned before, this is what the dysmorphologists I interviewed refer to as a *gestalt* moment: a moment of sudden recognition. And it is the moment when Dr Smith offers a diagnosis: 'We're talking about Kabuki'. Poppy has the nose but it is her mum that has the eyes and brow. So the defining features of Kabuki are seen in the juxtaposition of features distributed across the two bodies assumed to be biologically related. It is the juxtaposition of the slides of Poppy and her mother which evidences the syndrome. The team go on to discuss the significance of the case:

[Side profile of Poppy.]

DR MILNE: There aren't many [cases of Kabuki] across generations, Owen (another geneticist) has an unconfirmed one.

DR LITTLE: There is no actual report in the literature with a generational aspect [she adds that it would be a good case for someone to work up].

[Dr Smith briefly mentions a contact – her supervisor in the US who worked with the person who discovered or first wrote about Kabuki – to see if they are still doing work in this area. Dr Little doesn't pick this up.]

DR LITTLE: Mum's got the full house really.

DR MILNE: How about Manchester?

DR LITTLE: I think they've given up [doing work on this syndrome.]

[Slide of Mum's profile and hands.]

DR LITTLE: See the frontal finger pads and the tiny fifth finger ... can I take that to [London meeting of Dysmorphology Club]?

DR SMITH: Yes.

DR LITTLE: It's really helpful to see an adult, many die of renal failure, that's the worry. [She goes on to mention some of Mum's renal symptoms from the past for which she's had no treatment or examinations.] So that's a worry, so we need to look at her kidneys.

DR LITTLE: What's her IQ like?

DR LITTLE: Coping, just, in the 70s I think.

DR SMITH: They're a good family ... I can see if the Professor [Professor Kabuki] in Japan is still doing work in this area.

DR LITTLE: They would be a good family to do, Mum is so dramatic, I have no doubt in my mind.

[Dr Grey moves the slides on to a head and shoulders shot of a pretty young girl with blonde hair smiling into the camera.]

To make their portrait, the clinicians assemble slides of Poppy's face, hands and feet, and then juxtapose these with slides of her mother's face and hands. They make their readings of these features: that the toes are short, or that the eyes are slanting down, and align these with other materials they have collected and present as significant (such as a history of kidney disease, records of height measurements). They put all this together with records of Poppy's IQ and problems with her development (she's not coping at school even with help). The parts they are interested in are constituted as distinctive in terms of their shape and form (eyes, heads, toes, hands, fingers, nails, height), while Poppy's conduct is assessed against norms of intelligence and development. The implication is that her brain, like her hands, is malformed in some way.

The doctors are excited because the slide of Poppy's mother's face reveals a pattern across the representations, showing the defining features of Kabuki syndrome. In the case of Kabuki syndrome, which is rare, there is no so-called definitive or 'objective' evidence, i.e. no molecular test that confirms the clinical picture as the phenotypical expression of an aberrant genotype (cf. Kara *et al.* 2006). Therefore, I want to suggest that what is being implicitly performed here is not just the defining features of Kabuki, but rather, through the way in which the features are assembled and juxtaposed *across the bodies* of a mother and her

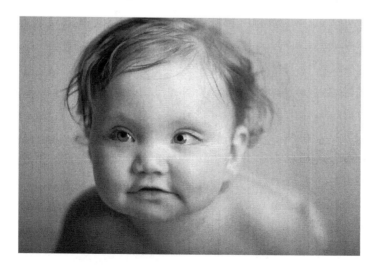

Figure 8.1 The face of Kabuki. Reproduced with kind permission of The Kabuki Syndrome Support Newtwork, http://kabukisyndrome.com/

child, it is being suggested that Kabuki is itself distributed across two biologically related bodies. This juxtaposition implies something pathological in common at the genetic level.

Constituting a relation between how Poppy and her mother look, the syndrome (Kabuki) and a genotype thus imply something more than the existence/presence of the syndrome itself. The portrait constructed of Poppy and her mother suggests that there is something shared at the genetic level, and (partially and provisionally) a possible syndrome–genotype relation, which cannot yet be made visible by molecular tests.

This is important, because most recorded cases of Kabuki are seen as sporadic, or de novo events. Familial cases fitting autosomal dominant inheritance have rarely been documented. I want to press, therefore, that the incompletion and provisionality of the portrait of Poppy and her biological relation is most important here: it gives opportunities for suggesting that which is not yet known and which cannot yet be fixed.

Portraying the genotype–phenotype (non-)relation

I am describing something very different here from the clinical process as portrayed in Mol's (2002) 'body multiple', where the clinic creates a perspective that coordinates all the fragments and heterogeneous parts into a hybrid, but settled and integrated, form, a diagnosis such as atherosclerosis of the lower leg. That form, as in Gilman's analysis mentioned above, settles into a single body, which can be taken to *represent* a disease category.

In contrast, in dysmorphology the heterogeneity and complexity does not always settle into the figure of an individual as being representative of a diagnosis. I am saying this despite the use of visual images of representative subjects in journal articles and websites, such as the figures of Sotos and Coffin-Lowry syndromes shown in earlier chapters. Contrastingly, the faces of Kabuki's representative subjects, and the more usual way of representing the face of a syndrome, can be seen in Figure 8.1. When the distributed nature of the phenotype *across* different bodies that are biologically related can be shown in the genetics clinic, then what is being revealed is that the genetic may be at work in producing the syndrome.

Dysmorphology's portraits thus conform in some ways to the science of visualizing disease mentioned earlier, and described so well by Gilman. However, there are differences of real significance in method and subject matter. The diverse visual and textual representations of *different* persons, their relations and their parts are assembled and juxtaposed: the features of a syndrome–genotype are not locatable in one body, in one individual, but across different bodies (see Figure 8.2 for an example). The syndrome (the phenotype) and its cause (an aberrant genotype) are distributed.

The complexity and heterogeneity of the defining features of a syndrome *need to be distributed* for them to stand as a phenotype, and the visible expression of the syndrome–genotype relation. Critically, what is implicit in these juxtapositions and in dysmorphologists' readings of them, is that there is something about the substance of the bodies of individuals that is not unique to them, but which is shared, or at least held in common to use Strathern's (2005) term. It is exceptionable that they are able to make the portraits show that it is not simply a disease that is shared, but rather that it is the common genetic substance, the genotype, that is pathological; and that the syndrome is the expression, or phenotype, of this common genotype, distributed across different bodies.

Therefore, the portrait in dysmorphology does not always reduce to the figure of an individual [as] a representative subject. Instead, it is the figure of a syndrome–genotype relation that emerges in the partial connection between the juxtaposition of materials deriving from different biologically realted bodies. I should stress, though, that juxtaposition here is not being made in the 'mode of comparison' (Strathern 1997): it is a different mode of ordering, one that flattens the world into divisions for a moment. Further, and this is important, what is being performed in the clinic is how the portrait makes a (temporary) space that cannot (yet) settle all the divisions and connections between all the parts across different bodies. And it is this distribution across different bodies that can be seen as the defining feature of dysmorphology's key portraits.

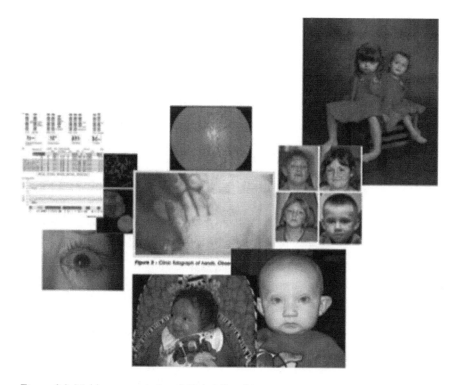

Figure 8.2 Making a portrait of Kabuki's phenotype–genotype relation. (Montage: Joanna Latimer)

Conclusion

The chapter has explained how the genetic clinic constructs clinical pictures as new forms of portraiture. Instead of showing individual figures in a pose that represents the features of a clinical diagnosis, dysmorphologists make *assemblages* of multiple and heterogeneous images of people's faces and their body parts, composed together with other visual materials, such as medical pedigrees, scans and tests results.

The method of assemblage and juxtaposition creates connections between the portraits and what it is that they seem to suggest. In my study of dysmorphology, it is the figure of a syndrome that is depicted by such assemblages. Although many assemblages remain in anticipation of such an outcome – the very possibility of defining the features of a syndrome–genotype relation is suggested by those moments when assemblages are drawn from biologically related bodies. In addition, I have shown how the juxtaposition of materials, such as the photographs of Poppy and her mother, can cast doubt on the significance of a test or report as well as be used as a method of confirmation or refutation.

What this form of portraiture performs, at one level, is the very possibility that the appearance of people's bodies and parts is the *expression* of a genotype. Clinicians' assemblages are made first to represent a phenotype or a syndrome, distributed across the substance of different persons and their parts. However, the geneticists use how the fleshy bodies look – the phenotype – to tell them about another and different kind of body – a genotype. How bodies across different persons 'look' is taken to mean something about the arrangement of genes. In this visualization and classification of the genetic, the clinic is ahead; laboratory-based science is lagging behind.

The ways in which features across families are juxtaposed also performs relations. Specifically, in my examination of dysmorphology's portraits, I have shown how the genetic clinic emerges as a space that gives *form* to the relation between genes (codes and information) and living, fleshy bodies. While 'morph' denotes shape, as I have already discussed, morphology is not just a branch of biology that deals with living forms; it is also a branch of grammar that deals with the formation and inflection of words. The two disciplines seem worlds apart, like the study of living forms and the 'post-genomic' representations of genes as information, codes and rules. Yet in a sense what dysmorphology's portraits do is to bring these worlds – the flesh and the grammar – into a relation because they help both *see* and *say* a genotype–syndrome relation.

The ways in which dysmorphology makes its portraits thus creates a space, a crossing, through which form is given to information (the aberrant genes), so that the gene is made visible. Here the gene is not only given presence, but is, for a moment, magnified. It is not simply, as Rabinow and Rose (2006) indicate in discussing the relation between the new genetics and strategies for the governing of life, that there is a very long chain of translation between the molecular and the molar – between information codes and the fleshy, vitality of the human organism. Rather, the molecular and the gene in models and in textual discourse mimic or simulate digital machines, and are performed as being of a different texture to fleshy bodies. As such, the molecular gene brings with it a different, incompatible world to that which is occupied by fleshy, living bodies: these two worlds seem irreducible, they are in a *non-relation* (Foucault 1983).

For all this, as this chapter has demonstrated, the transition from a world of flesh to a world of texts and surfaces is hardly as complete as Haraway fears. For the moment, the clinic is precisely a key *site* in which crossings between these two worlds can happen. This is partly because of what the clinic makes its composites of the organic and inorganic mean in terms of genes, but it is also because of how medicine performs representations *as* reality.

Hence I also want to press the kind of scientific work being enacted here: assemblage and juxtaposition is a mode suited to a correlational science looking to take forward *classification*, rather than being compatible to an experimental science seeking causes. What I suggest these methods of portraiture both reflect and constitute is the shift in genetic science from one gene as responsible for one disease, to the complexity of classifying a syndrome–phenotype as the expression of a genotype. Thus, the portrait is a way of representing syndromes that does not reduce them either to a single gene or to the figure of an individual and, instead, allows syndromes to emerge in the partial connection between the assemblage and juxtaposition of materials deriving from different, biologically related bodies. In this we can see how the clinic is doing the '*new* genetics'. I discuss the significance of these aspects of the study further in Chapter 12.

Part IV
The family and identities

9   Genes, bodies, persons

Perhaps the individual is so viable a god because he can actually understand the ceremonial significance of the way he is treated, and quite on his own can respond dramatically to what is proffered him. In contacts between such deities there is no need for middlemen; each of these gods is able to serve as his own priest.

(Goffman 2005, p.95)

Introduction

In the previous chapter I have shown how the method of assemblage and juxta-position in dysmorphology – what I am calling their portraits – enacts the clinic as making syndromes visible as an effect of a phenotype–genotype relation. This means that the clinic, through its immersion in the fleshy world of the family, can make visible what the laboratory cannot, *as yet*. This is because the clinic is a site of crossing between two incompatible worlds, namely that of information and codes – the genotype – and that of the flesh and social interaction – the phenotype.

We have seen how the dysmorphology clinic accomplishes this crossing of worlds through shifting between its front stage, where it enacts itself at the white-board as scientific, and its backstage, with its immersion in the fleshy, messy world of people, families, and bodies. Questions arise, therefore, as to what persons become in the clinical processes that help rebirth the clinic. Are they more or less molecularized in the form of the distributed effects of their DNA? And, if so, what happens to them as individual subjects, the individual god-like creature described by Goffman (2005, p.95) above?

Debates on the new genetics, together with ongoing developments in biologi-cal theory, appear to rewrite the body, undermining not only the figure of the individual but challenging ideas of what it is to be human. As I have begun to suggest in the previous chapter, recent writing suggests that the new genetics, particularly molecular biology, and its implications for how we think the body and persons, signals an era of the 'posthuman'. This is due in part to the way the new genetics, or 'postmodern biology' (Melley 2002, p.51), appears to trouble body–self relations.

Specifically, commentators suggest that a 'geneticization' of the body could provoke a revolution in our ways of conceiving persons as individual, and lead to the destruction of the human:

> What is the posthuman? Think of it as a point of view characterised by the following assumptions … First, the posthuman view privileges informational pattern over material instantiation, so that embodiment in biological substrate is seen as an accident of history rather than an inevitability of life. Second, the posthuman view considers consciousness, regarded as the seat of human identity in the Western tradition long before Descartes thought he was a mind thinking, as an epiphenomenon, as an evolutionary upstart trying to claim that it is the whole show when in actuality it is only a minor side show. Third, the posthuman view thinks of the body as the original prosthesis we all learn to manipulate, so that extending or replacing the body with other prostheses becomes a continuation of a process that began before we were born.
>
> (Hayles 1999, pp.2–3)

Hayles is suggesting that the shift to molecular biology heralds the destruction of the human because there is an undermining of the three pillars that underpin human exceptionalism: the uniqueness of the body–individual, the supremacy of consciousness and the human/other dualism.

However, as I have indicated in Chapter 2, medicine has many more associations (and much more at stake in how it maintains its dominant position) than its attachment to either biology or science. Specifically, as I illustrate in the following two chapters, these associations are with society and the family. Ahead of this, however, I am suggesting that one of medicine's crucial attachments is to the other humanist ideas that run alongside those of science, especially those of welfare and justice.

In the rest of this chapter I hold the clinical practices in dysmorphology against the more general ideas underpinning debate on the geneticization of the body, in order to challenge presumptions that the figure of the individual is disappearing. I begin by examining research that suggests that the new genetics may be rewriting the relation between bodies and selves to deconstruct the figure of the individual. I go on to show how medicine in the genetic clinic holds two apparently contradictory notions over bodies and persons in play, before exploring what this helps accomplish.

Re-writing the individual?

I am reflecting on Foucault's examination of the way in which the clinic as a social institution is central to the apparatus of nation states that allows for the protection, as well as the enhancement, of people and their bodies (see also Hewitt 1983). There has been a great deal of critique of the clinic as a site in which the person as a social being is abstracted, or that the clinic is often seen as a space that institutes the mind/body split. Similarly, many think of it as a space which helps organize the division between the medical body and the lived body in such a way as to exclude personhood, and particular ways of thinking and knowing the body and its troubles.

Less of a focus, however, has been the way the clinic, in performing these divisions, also performs a key duality inherent in the humanist tradition, which is linked to the compound figure of the individual of humanist thought. Within this latter perspective, the clinic has long been understood as a site constitutive of the dominant body–self relations that underpin modern biopolitics (see also Latimer 2013). Foucault (2003a, 2003b) and Deleuze (1997) among others have precisely connected the operations of clinical power to ideas of the integrated, discrete body–self. Specifically, each has shown how modern politics works consciousness through the body, both the substantial body *and* the body as an idea. They have also explored how the clinic has been pivotal to establishing this biopolitics of the body. For example, the clinic has helped to constitute how we think of the body, and the ways in which we think the body circulates ideas of the normal, the individual, and individual–society relations.

Any new ways of thinking about the body's basic fabric and functions, such as growth and development, that erodes notions of persons as individual would, therefore, have profound implications for ways of ordering social relations. As Strathern (2006) stresses:

> Bodily uniqueness is a sign, as much as it is a Euro-American symbol, of autonomy and respect for the person as an individual ... but genes are not unique at all – the combination might be unique but the genes are replicas.
>
> (pp.20–1)

Hence, while the destruction of the human figure represents for some a potentially liberating ontology of connectivity, there are profound implications for humanist traditions of welfare and justice. Habermas (2003) questions the decoupling of a specifically human nature, not least because of its consequences for the functioning of the many social institutions that rely on notions of individual responsibility, conscience, will, and so forth.

This analysis involves my returning to dysmorphology's portraits to examine the kinds of bodies and persons that they perform. Chapter 8 showed how the genetic clinic constructs clinical pictures of syndromes as new forms of portraiture: assemblages in which multiple and heterogeneous images of biologically related bodies and their parts are juxtaposed. As might be expected, these portraits, through particular modes of representing, reconfigure people and their parts as the visible, momentary expression of a genotype as the origin of a syndrome. Yet this is not to say that all aspects of *personhood* are so encapsulated. Instead, as I am about to show in the current chapter, what stands out are shifts in ground that perform persons as at one moment unique and at another as made up of substance that is shared, or, as Strathern (2006) puts it, held in *common* with others.

Deconstructing the human?

Many writers have been at pains to show how the revolution in biology offers new forms of classification and categorization, which may or may not break down some of the old classificatory divisions (Rabinow 1992, 1996). Here there are arguments that this revolution does not just lead us back to old forms of biological determinism, or the Cartesian mind/body split. Rather, by offering individual genetic profiles that are also located in a collective gene pool (Flower and Heath 1993) geneticization of the body may characterize a 'recombinant bio-politics' (Dillon and Read 2001) that unpicks the fundamental principles of humanism and the polarity of individual/population that underpins the ordering of social relations.

In contrast, for many years sociologists have been attempting to 'bring back the body' (Frank 1990), an agenda which has involved deconstructing ideas of persons that previously kept in play the mind/body split. Consequently, the incorporation of phenomenological traditions has introduced an alternative to the objectification of the body found in medicine, and helped to reinstate an idea of the body as 'lived' (Leder 1990), both as the realm of the self (Young 1997) and of individuals as 'body-persons' (Latimer 2009a). What has been instituted in this emergent tradition on embodiment is an idea of the body not just as a site of inscription and disciplinary effects (Brush 1998), including the institution of particular subjectivities (Biehl and Moran-Thomas 2009) or even of the importance of embodiment in acculturation and social ordering (Bourdieu 1977; Mauss 1973). In their place people emerge as bodies, both with as well as without organs (Deleuze and Guattari 1987), as fleshy and yet as more than flesh (Fox 2012).

An emergent body of research is also exploring the cultural, political and social significance of the way that bodies and persons are performed by the practices, artefacts and discourses of medicine at the interface with the new genetics and reproductive technologies (e.g. Atkinson *et al.* 2006; Brodwin 2002; Carsten 2004; Clarke 1998; Clarke *et al.* 2010; Martin 1991; Pálsson 2007; Thompson 2005). Theorists have sought to identify the new *identities* flowing from the revolution in genetic medicine and technoscience – such as 'carriers', 'prepatients', 'surrogate' mothers and fathers, 'somatic citizens', and so on and so forth.

Within this tradition, feminist science and technology studies and cultural studies scholars, as well as medical anthropologists, are exploring how changes in biomedical understandings of the body may not be just changing disease categories or constituting new identities, but may make explicit new ontologies, particularly of connectivity. This is not to suggest that human materiality, for example DNA, determines human nature. Rather, it is to explore how discoveries in molecular biology incorporated into clinical science can undo the very body–self relations that underpin so much of Western thought. Let me elaborate.

Emergent understandings from the biosciences have the possibility of changing perceptions of the body, and thereby of the existence of human beings. Contemporary discoveries seem to suggest that bodies are not, as previously understood, bounded, contained, homogeneous, fixed and integrated entities.

Rather new thinking in molecular biology seems to trouble the self/not-self division that is the defining feature performed by the figure of the individual body. This can be understood in several ways.

Firstly, as Haraway (2007) points out, human bodies are not made up of uniquely human substance, but are themselves heterogeneous:

> I love the fact that human genomes can be found in only about 10% of the cells that occupy the mundane space I call my body; the other 90% of the cells are filled with genomes of bacteria, fungi, protists, and such, some of which play in a Symphony necessary to my being alive at all, and some of which are hitching a ride and doing the rest of me, of us, no harm ... To be one is always to be many.
>
> (pp.3–4)

The new genetics thus puts into play an idea that '[w]ithin "us" is the most threatening other – the propagules,[1] whose phenotype we temporarily are' (Haraway 1991, p.217).

Secondly, breakthroughs made possible because of new genetic technoscience offer ways of rethinking body–persons as made up of substance from a much wider gene pool, and of the body as the temporary and partial expression of a genotype. Within this perspective it is the DNA that is immortal, and the genes that are the 'time travellers', while the body or soma is just the transport vehicle, which like a 'hired car', is the temporary and dispensable host for their reproduction (Olshansky and Carnes 2001).

Living in the parts of others

It seems from the preceding discussion that the new genetics has the potential to destroy the usual image of the individual that, as Strathern (1992a) has illuminated, is *the* trope performed by Euro-American, modernist ideas of kinship:

> A child was endowed with material from both parents, literally formed from parts of them. Yet it was regarded as equivalent to neither mother or father nor to the relation between them: rather it was a hybrid product in another sense, a genetically unique individual with a life of its own. It was only a part of their life, despite the fact that its genetic material was formed wholly of theirs.
>
> (pp.93–4)

As Melley (2002) discussing Haraway points out, this is partly because of how postmodern biology 'privileges "biotic components" over the "traditional organism" (p.50). Instead of the '"single unit of masterly control", what appears is a new kind of biological organism that is a "pastiche of multiple centres and peripheries"' (pp.50–1).

Melley goes on to show how, within this perspective, the apparent unravelling of the body–self as unique and individuated is specifically being done by 'nature' and the materiality of bodies 'talking back' in surprising ways, so that postmodern biology is forcing (humanist) social philosophy to re-theorize, particularly over notions of the agentic subject and the possessive individual.

Martin (2010), for example, in her work on microchimerism and 'cell trafficking' between mother and foetus suggests that, in the history of microchimerism, biomedical scientists have had to struggle with an anomaly that undoes the metaphor of the bounded, individual body–self that forms the basis of immunology theory:

> In microchimeric bodies, cells that are coded as 'not-self' are living and reproducing happily in body-nations that are not their 'own'. In this way, ontologies are shifting in light of the unexpected, as are appropriate metaphors of what the biological (and indeed social) 'self' is.
>
> (p.25)

What happens in immunology is that this surprise finding about 'fetal' cells living in the 'motherland' (the body of the mother) challenges the underpinning ideas of bodies, persons, and the immune system based on the self/not-self division: immunology relies on an understanding of bodily substance (cells) of persons as being a territory that is uniquely their own.

What Martin proposes is that emergent understandings have the potential to shift the model of the fetus as foreign, to a model that recasts the maternal–fetal relationship in ways that blur the borders of bodies so that individuals reemerge not as discrete and unique, but as 'constitutively intermingled' (p.26). Following Douglas's (2003) emphasis on the mirroring of the fleshy and the social body, Martin explores how the migratory character of globalization mirrors this intermingling to trouble the bordering that underpins the politics of nation-states.

Critically, if the heterogeneous nature of a human being's substance is unmasked as not entirely their own (or even as all human), it becomes harder to resettle them into the figure of the unique individual (see also Latimer 2009b). Specifically, is this an 'ontic politics' (Verran 2011) in which understandings from the new genetics might help in the process of unpicking the ideas that bind the body to the figure of the possessive, autonomous individual and the dominant power relations that flow from this binding?

If so, questions also arise as to what then happens to persons if the figure of the individual is first deconstructed, and then reconfigured as the constituents of a phenotype. We must ask whether this partial phenotype is merely the material expression of an informational pattern, a genotype, made up of elements of information coming from a gene pool that is common to many, even non-human, others.

Bodies in dysmorphology

As already discussed, questions arise over what kinds of body–persons get produced and reproduced in the relationship between geneticization processes, the clinic, the body, and cultural conceptions of personhood. In Chapter 8 I have suggested that dysmorphology's portraits conform in some ways to the science of visualizing disease, but that there are differences of real significance in method and subject matter. The various visual and textual representations of different persons, their relations, and their parts, are assembled and juxtaposed: the features of a syndrome–genotype are not locatable in one body, in one individual, but across different bodies. The syndrome and its cause (an aberrant phenotype) are distributed.

In dysmorphology, heterogeneity and complexity do not always settle into the figure of an individual as 'representative' of a diagnosis. Rather it reflects and consitutues the shift in genetic science from one gene as responsible for one disease (the OGOD syndrome of media hype mentioned in Chapter 1), to the complexity of a syndrome–phenotype relation that may represent a genotype. Thus, the portrait in dysmorphology, such as the one of Kabuki presented in Chapter 8 offers the figure of a syndrome–genotype relation. This does not reduce either to a single gene or to the figure of an individual and, instead, emerges in its partial connection between the assemblage and juxtaposition of materials deriving from different bodies. The portrait in the clinic makes a (temporary) space that cannot (yet) settle all the division and connections between all the parts across different bodies. And it is this distribution and deferral that is the defining feature of some of dysmorphology's key portraits. The complexity and heterogeneity of the defining features of a syndrome *need to be distributed* for them to stand as a phenotype, and so act as the visible expression of the syndrome–genotype relation. As I have said at the end of Chapter 8, this is the clinic doing the 'new' as opposed to the 'old' genetics.

Bringing back family

In conducting the above analysis, I have suggested that dysmorphology's portraits help make information flesh, and flesh into information. So much so that the clinic itself becomes the crossing, the bridge, the interdisciplinary site through which the word gets made flesh. I want now to return to the dysmorphologists' discourse to unpack how persons are being represented.

In the interview with Professor Smart he describes a case that was referred to him. As he talks to me he is showing me photographs and images on his laptop and recalling his meeting with a family:

PROFESSOR SMART: ... this was a really surprising case to us. This little girl here [shows me a photograph on his laptop of a small girl], we got the referral letter from a dermatologist saying 'Please see this girl because Mum says she's got little patches, tiny patches of hairiness on her, and we don't know what it is'. We didn't know what we'd got to expect. So here she is, [shows me another photo of the girl on his laptop] she comes into clinic. *She is a normal little girl* and these are the little patches of hair [points to the patches of hair on the little girl in the photo], first I'm thinking 'she's a very fussy mother', you can hardly see them, do you see what I mean? Then this is where you've got to know a bit of dysmorphology. She has got a big head, okay, a significantly big head *even though she is normal*, but right on the top of the range [size of head for age], hairy patches on the skin, big head, whatever. There is something called Gorlin syndrome. Now Gorlin syndrome is caused *by a dominant gene*, and it is a funny syndrome. If you've got the gene you don't get hairy patches funnily enough, but you do get a big head and you get a tendency towards what are called basal cell carcinomas – which are actually skin cancers – and you get other things with a tendency to dural cysts as well. So actually we asked if anybody had any tooth/jaw problems – Dad said 'yes, I had a jaw cyst, when I was a child' – and he had a big head as well.

JL: This is the dad? [Photo of a man's head now displayed on the laptop.]

PROFESSOR SMART: The dad. So then you've got to know a bit more dysmorphology – because what else can you look for in the dad? Well they [people with Gorlin syndrome] have – if you x-ray their chest, they can have cysts in the ribs, and if you've x-rayed their skull they can have some cysts in the skull – but they also have these little pits on their hands – I can show you a picture, I thought I had, there you are [shifts to a picture of a man's hands] – if you look at that palm, you can see these little tiny pits – that's Dad's palm – so all that from a child that has come in with a little patch of hair, and what we thought might have been a fussy mother, we made a diagnosis – because Dad didn't know that he had this. So he has got a tendency to skin cancer, which is worth knowing about, and I guess it is worth knowing about for the child as well. So if somebody writes it up – hairy patches as a possible feature of Gorlin syndrome, then of course everybody will start to look and then somebody will write another paper saying that we know what to look for now.

In this extract Professor Smart helps us to see how dysmorphology constructs its clinical pictures through assembling and juxtaposing parts of persons drawn from across the family – the little girl's hairy patches and big head, and the father's big head, history (jaw cyst) and the scans of his bones. The clinical picture is a portrait of Gorlin syndrome – which is known to be an effect of a dominant gene and is an inherited condition.

In this rendering, then, for a moment the little girl and her father become a phenotypical expression of what is going on at the genetic level. In the portrait in dysmorphology, such as the one of Gorlin being represented by Professor Smart, the figure of a phenotype–genotype relation emerges in the partial connection between the assemblage and juxtaposition of materials deriving from different bodies. In the clinic the portrait makes a (temporary) space that cannot (yet) settle all the division and connections between all the parts across different bodies. And it is this that is, as I have already suggested in the previous chapter, the defining feature of some of dysmorphology's portraits. The complexity and heterogeneity of the defining features of a syndrome *need to be distributed* across the bodies of people who are biologically related for them to stand as a phenotype, and the visible expression of a phenotype–genotype relation.

However, what is implicit in these juxtapositions and dysmorphologists' readings of them is that there is something about the substance of individuals' bodies that is not unique to them, but is 'held in common' (Strathern 2006). Making the portraits show that it is not simply a disease that is distributed across different biologically related bodies, but the patterns of unusual or pathological features that are distributed is of significance. This is because it suggests that the patterns are the effects, or expression, of a common genetic substance, the genotype.

In accomplishing this, dysmorphology's portraits help make information flesh, and turn flesh into information: so that the clinic becomes the crossing, the cross-disciplinary site through which the informational codes (genes) get made flesh. And at these moments we can see a geneticization of the body, and the destruction of the figure of the individual. Hence, dysmorphology process seems, on occasion, to efface those body–self relations that are performed by the figure of the individual and that underpin modernity.

However, gene medicine would be nothing if it were only concerned with people as dehumanized – as biologically determined effects, made up of informational fragments coming from a gene pool; as if the body–person were merely a temporary home for DNA that will be passed on ('reshuffled', as Olshansky and Carnes (2001) put it) to take shape in other forms down the line. Dysmorphology's portraits instead perform the idea that it is the syndrome–genotype that is made of distributed fragments, not persons. In making this move, the clinic affords a space for bringing back persons (rather than bodies) in ways that rescue them from the destructive effects of the genetic, both in terms of the symbolic violence of a totalizing geneticization of the body, and in terms of the literal and fleshy effects of a genetic aberration.

Specifically, as Professor Smart makes his portrait of a potential new discovery in the natural history of Gorlin syndrome, he switches between portraying the little girl and her father as phenotypes (as mere distributed parts that signify a syndrome and that express a genotype), and personifying the little girl and her father *as persons*. This switch is implicit in his account: '...because Dad didn't know that he had this. So he [Dad] has got a tendency to skin cancer, which is worth knowing about, and I guess it is worth knowing about for the child as well'.

In his deft account of the dad and the little girl's need for knowledge about their bodies being at risk of cancer, Professor Smart invokes the figure of these two people as persons with needs of a very particular kind – as in need of knowledge. This is an example of what Strathern (2009) illuminates as a very contemporary Euro-American rendering of enlightenment personhood: namely that a context (the science) that gives people better knowledge and understanding of their bodies will then help them make choices and exert their autonomous decision-making.

By refiguring them as persons who need knowledge *about* their bodies, Professor Smart gives the man and his daughter presence *as* Euro-American persons. In doing so he refigures the daughter and the father as human in this very special sense: as people with bodies and as people who can know about their bodies in order to act differently. That is, he refigures them in terms of the Cartesian legend: as capable of thought elevated over the body. For a moment, then, the little girl and her father are not just figured as the effects of their aberrant genes, as informational codes distributed across the bodies of different persons. These kinds of moves put into play a *need to know* that happens over and over again; for example, we can hear it in the discussion of Poppy and her mother analysed in the previous chapter.

In addition, as he gives his account, Professor Smart also refigures himself as not just concerned with knowledge about genes and syndromes, but as working in the institution of medicine that is heroic and humanist. This is because his discourse makes present how his work helps with the saving of lives and the prevention of unnecessary suffering – in this case cancer. In order to make this switch in ground, to move from the importance of the medical gaze to the welfare of persons, he is also aligning his gaze with a humanist ethics. Professor Smart is giving an account that, as at the same time as it justifies the clinical science, it also refigures patients as more than clinical objects: it reattaches him, and the clinic, to the girl and her dad as both persons *and* as the ultimate source of knowledge.

I want to emphasize that this switch in alignment – from genes, and their expression, to the frailty of flesh, and to the potential for suffering – moves its speaker between two contrasting moral imperatives both of which can be addressed by knowledge. This is medicine's 'godtrick'. Not just to perform an epistemology–ontology relation able to read the book of nature, in this case the genotype–phenotype that produces a syndrome, but also to be in alignment with a moral universe that conjoins knowledge (information) to the relief of suffering and the support of a world of choice and autonomy.

Recovering the human

Through such switches in alignment the human seemingly gets recovered. Together, clinicians and parents bring into play many different ways of giving each other presence as human beings. For example, as I have already indicated in Chapter 6, clinicians do not just have to pass as experts with a special gaze; in their interactions with the family and with the children, they must also personify themselves as fellow humans. In consequence, in order for their gaze to pass in both forms of membership, clinicians have to become *motile*.

We heard some of this complexity in Professor Fox's description of her practice discussed in Chapter 6, but what also emerged through this description is how, in expressing her own need to appear as nice, Professor Fox is giving the baby and the parents presence as human beings. Thus at one moment in their alignment with the gene, clinicians perform a detachment, a gaze, that constructs portraits of children and their families that can be made to represent a syndrome, and in the suggestion of substance in common, a syndrome–genotype relation. But at other moments dysmorphologists do more than this: they reinstate the family members as persons, as much *more than the sum of their bodily parts*.

In the following extract the clinicians are discussing a child who has just left the clinic: David, an 8-year-old boy with seizures, motor problems and severe developmental delay. Here, even in the case of a syndrome that is so very pervasive across systems, David is reclaimed as a person who is both an effect of and yet as more than his genotype:

DR SMITH (CG): Isn't he lovely?
DR JONES (SPR): Fab, you just get glimpses …
DR SMITH: … of what he could be like. Do you think he'll ever speak?
DR JONES: *No. He can communicate though. He has a good understanding of how the world works and how to get people to do what he wants.*
DR SMITH: The majority of kids with polymicrogyria are very happy children.
DR JONES: So chromosomes 21 and 22.
DR SMITH: Yes, I expect them to be normal but worth looking for. There's one X-linked gene where they have narrowed down where it could be, that will be interesting for him, he fits that mould. It would be useful for the daughter, and people like to know why.
DR PARRY (SPR): If they don't find it they are chasing rainbows.
[Dr Smith goes on to explain David as a 'classic polymicrogyria' – dribbling, gait, no speech, developmental problems, coordination problems, epilepsy.]
(Emphasis added)

Sometimes, we are told, you 'just get glimpses' of what David 'could be like'. As a 'normal', lovely child living a happy family life. He fits the mould of an X-linked genetic problem, and he is a classic case of polymicrogyria. Yet David, after all, can transcend his bodiedness, because he is refigured for a moment as having consciousness, he'll never speak but: 'He can communicate though. He has a good understanding of how the world works and how to get people to do what he wants.'

While a child may be 'effaced' (Bauman 1990) by the genetic, the actors responsible for them – the clinicians and the parents – are not effacing their humanity even as they also constitute their abnormality. It is the syndrome–genotype that effaces the face of a child. Here I am thinking of how the child as 'the face of the *Other* ... as an authority *without force*' (Bauman 1989, p.214, my emphasis) could be, in these situations, effaced. Their 'face' as the most delicate of interaction's effects (Black 2011; Goffman 1999, 2005) could also be obliterated, to figure them as less than human. However, while dysmorphologists read the faces of children as objects and expressions of a syndrome, through the moves that we have seen in this chapter they reinstate the child, erasing their Otherness, to refold them in the category of the human, and as in need of protection and love. This means that at the same time as clinicians draw upon a notion that the child's condition is biologically determined, rather than socially or culturally conditioned, they hold to an idea that there is an essence to persons: that people have a real nature, and that each child is unique and essentially human. This occurs, despite abnormalities of appearances, despite appearances on the surface and 'essences' thought to exist in the depths of the body.

In these ways the integral, discrete body is what helps to create the figure of the individual. Critically though, in order to be seen as *truly* human and so transcend their bodiedness the individual must also be able to 'disembody'. It is in this last respect, distinguished by the observation of his consciousness, that David is reaffirmed as human, as having face, and as much more than the sum of his bodily parts, common or not.

The double figure

The current chapter has examined not only when geneticization of the body is in play in the practices of the clinic, but also when it is not. The focus has been on how the clinic (and the production and reproduction of body–persons enacted through clinical practices) acts as one site in which cultural conceptions of what it is to be human are instituted in a post-genomic era. As has been seen, the clinic switches alignment from the gene to the family, to keep other ways of thinking about the human, and persons, in play.

The 'defining feature' of humanist thought, to draw on Jordonova's (2000) productively ambiguous phrase about portraits, is the double figure of an individual consciousness incarnated within its own distinctive and recognizable corporeality. At one moment a person is deeply connected to enlightenment ideas of their human nature being individuated, one that involves the possibility of agency, responsibility, autonomy, subjectivity and choice (Strathern 1988, 1991, 1992a, 2006). At other moments it is their corporeality that makes them distinctive and can set them apart.

The relation between the integral, contained, corporeal body and that of the autonomous individual helps perform the figure of the human. This figure of the human is the cultural icon that underpins most contemporary forms of social organization in the West, including sociological theory itself (Skeggs 2004, 2011; Strathern 2006). But alongside this idea of the individuated body–self runs the paradoxical and parallel seam of Western thought that detaches rationality from the body: the individual, at moments of choice and autonomous decision-making, has to be rational. They must have knowledge from a singular, undivided perspective, a perspective that stands outside the plane of personal (that is bodily) action (Latimer 2007a; Strathern 1992a).

Against notions of the integral, contained body, individuals to be fully human also have to demonstrate a capacity for detachment. To attain the singular perspective of rationality, man[2] must be able to *disembody*:

> Many features of contemporary knowledges – knowledges based on the presumption of a singular reality, pre-existent representational categories, and an unambiguous terminology able to be produced and utilized by a singular, rational, and unified knowing subject who is unhampered by personal 'concerns' – can be linked to man's disembodiment, his detachment from his manliness in producing knowledge or truth.
>
> (Grosz 1993, p.205)

Paradoxically, it is the conjoined figure of the person as integral body *and* a unique discrete consciousness that helps to portray the individual as human. To be fully human, and transcend their bodiedness, the individual must be able to detach rather than simply 'disembody' as many have read Descartes (Foucault 1979a). Yes, it is a capacity to transcend the body that distinguishes humanity from its animality, but, in the Western tradition, it is nonetheless the *detachment* of consciousness that remains the defining feature of human exceptionalism and potency.[3]

The human, once distinguished by this detachment of consciousness, is thus able to settle into a complex whole. Curiously it is not the envelope of the body, its form, that can be caught in paint or in a photograph, so much as it is a detachment of consciousness from bodily experiences that defines the individual. Yes, representations of the corporeal body must take up most of the painting, photograph or sculpture, but it is the capture of the character (the eyes, stance and gesture) that enlivens the flesh and makes these more than a representation of a corpse. To be seen as human, persons must exhibit characteristics, such as willpower, desire, vulnerability, or moral strength.

At moments clinicians bring into play grounds that displace bodily biology as that which both determines personhood, and re*affirms* a child's humanity, as well as their own.[4] Put simply, clinicians circulate that crucial move in humanist thought: the moment when the figure of the individual is performed as transcending their bodiedness. In other words, in the clinic grounds are made available through which people such as David can be figured *as* human, because they are much more than the sum of their bodily parts. At other times, however much they protect the humanity of the present child, clinicians will not hesitate to agree that reproducing such a child would be better avoided. That is why the doctor mentions that David's sister needs to know more about his diagnosis, in case it has implications for her own reproductive future.

Reaffirming medicine's humanism

As detailed in Chapter 8, the genetic clinic constructs clinical pictures as new forms of portraiture: assemblages in which multiple and heterogeneous images of different people's bodies and parts of their bodies are juxtaposed. These new forms of portraiture reflect and help constitute the new genetics. However, rather than these portraits making the distributed and hybrid nature of *personhood* explicit, shifts in ground mean that what is being portrayed is the figure of a syndrome, and the possibility of defining the features of a *syndrome–genotype* relation. Within the perspective provided by the alignment of the clinic and the new genetics, the bodies of children and their biological relations – ever more anatomized – are fragmented into objects, and made to represent a syndrome, or even, where possible, a genotype.

Geneticization of the body at these moments thus risks not so much deconstructing the human as destroying this central trope of society – thus setting back the more sociologically acceptable ways of deconstructing the 18th century notions of the individual we have inherited. Yet, at the same time, the clinic still keeps in play an idea that people – like the boy David but unlike their bodies – are *much more than the sum of their parts*. Specifically, all the parts that make up the body of the person can still be transcended at moments to refigure the human: the complex individual of humanist thought.

This is important because, as Haraway (2007) reminds us, the humanist production of the individual includes notions of human rights that are critical to social justice, which can help rescue those categories of persons at risk of social exclusion, marginalization and violence. As it happens, the double figure of the human brought into play within the clinic protects against individuals like David being constituted as non-human enough to become what Haraway describes as 'killable'.[5] Portraiture thus affords the clinic more than its ability to detect the origins of the form of bodies and their parts – and all their concomitant troubles – from their appearance: it also helps to remind us that appearances are, after all, deceiving. As Marx notes, 'If the essence and appearance of things directly coincided, all science would be superfluous' (1991, p.956).

Alongside its on-going engagement with the posthuman, the clinic reinvigorates itself simultaneously as a protagonist of the human. It is this motility, the capacity of clinicians to switch grounds, which helps medicine reinvigorate its place as what Foucault (2003a) described as the queen of the *human* sciences rather than the *life* sciences. Even in genetic science's alignment with the new genetics, medical advances in this field offer different ways to see the body. In doing so, medicine revives the notion that persons are much more than simply determined by their biology.

This accepted, the figure of the human being produced and reproduced in the clinic remains a vision of the individual agentic self, distinctive by a form of consciousness that can transcend its bodiedness and so detach itself. In other words, this is not a relational kind of personhood, a vision of 'dividual' persons as the creations of the relations that make them up (Latimer 2009b drawing on Strathern 1988). Rather, the clinic in dysmorphology still gives presence to the compound figure of the individual of humanist thought, such as that portrayed by Rodin in his sculpture *The Thinker*.

Conclusion

In this chapter I have explored the interaction of genetic science, the clinic and Euro-American conceptions of personhood, and I have discussed how there is debate in the social sciences about the way the new genetics is changing ideas of what it is to be human. This is particularly apparent in the way commentators predict that 'geneticization' rewrites the body.

Inasmuch as it lead towards a revolution in our ways of conceiving persons, this rewriting of the body is said to hold possibilities for the decoupling of the fundamental principles of humanism and the polarity of individual/population that underpins the ordering of social relations. Specifically, there are notions abroad that the new genetics undermines the very ideas that underpin modernity: such as the figure of the integrated discrete individual body/self.

I have held these various ideas against the practices of genetic medicine. Against a straightforward geneticization of the body, including the undermining of the figure of the individual, I have shown how medicine in the clinic does not necessarily exclude but rather helps maintain the availability of some crucial and basic tenets of enlightenment humanism. Surprisingly, perhaps, the alignment of the new genetics and the clinic may well be extending possibilities for performances of the human.

Specifically, switches in alignment afford the clinic moments for the performance of persons as capable of transcending their bodies, despite their genes. It is not just that the various parts get reconciled into a whole – the figure of the individual as the basis of humanist thought and contemporary forms of governing. Rather, at moments, the clinic reasserts how all the parts that make up the body of the person can still be transcended, in order to refigure the Cartesian mind–body relation. It is this switch in ground that helps medicine reinstate its position as the guardian of the complex individual of humanist thought that underpins notions of welfare, respect and justice.

What I want to emphasize, for the purposes of the present chapter, is that at the very moment that children such as David are reaffirmed and given shelter in the fold of the human, their difference is also being denied. In doing this, the doctors may be understood as reaffirming themselves as more complex humans – as able one moment to 'attach' to others and in another to 'detach' from them in order to read the book of nature. As such, the clinic becomes a site that switches between the objectivity of scientific gaze and a kind of banal phenomenology of the subject, which denies particular forms of life and relationality, and particular ways of being and becoming.

In summary, the analysis I have presented so far does more than problematize existing conceptions about how medicine is being geneticized. It also helps us to see how medicine switches its extensions and attachments: at one moment it performs the gaze as a pure, detached, clinical moment, as processes through which people and their parts are objectified; in the next it reattaches to the complex individuals of humanist thought. In making these switches, medicine not only reinvigorates itself as the protagonist of the human but, as is discussed in the next two chapters, extends its colonization of the family and what Ginsburg and Rapp (1991) call the 'politics of reproduction'.

10 'The family' and medicine

Whether primacy is given to social ties or biological ones, it seems that the late twentieth century affords new possibilities for people who wish to be certain about how and why they are related. This is true of both legal redress (what the courts will countenance) and of technological intervention in the reproductive process. As possibilities, these instruments and techniques exist in a cultural environment of empowerment or enablement.

(Strathern 1996, p.37)

Choice has become the privileged vantage from which to measure all action.

(Strathern 1992c, p.36)

Introduction

In previous chapters I have shown how dysmorphology combines classical approaches to medical diagnosis with methods of genetic profiling (including molecular tests) in order to differentiate the normal from the abnormal, and the genetic from the non-genetic. In this chapter, I review the relationship of medicine and the family against a background of discourses of child development.

An entangling of family in discourses of health and consumption has instituted parenting as a specific site of identity-work. So much so that 'parenting' emerges as being a qualitatively different experience from being either a mother or father. I illustrate how the bodies of children have become the visible manifestation and measure of 'good' parenting within these discourses, both in terms of children looking 'good' (in a double sense – as of aesthetic and moral value), and looking healthy. My aim is to show how these aspects of good parenting are prefigured by a consumer culture with an emphasis on 'lifestyle choice'.

Contrastingly, at the same time as the alignment of the clinic with the family intensifies the responsibalization of parents as reproducing the future of healthy progeny, it also helps to institute parents as more than agents providing the right kind of environment for their child. Significantly, it treats them as *biological beings* whose substance may be problematic, particularly in the context of reproduction.

In what follows, therefore, I explore how the dysmorphology clinic specifically stands at the intersection of genetic technoscience, the family and persons. Critically, I argue that this intersection sets up an intimate involvement with the family that helps produce new forms of identity for parents on the one hand, including figuring people (parents, children and siblings) as 'future parents', and enables dysmorphology to hold its special place in genetic science on the other.

The family and public health

It is well rehearsed that the clinic has been critical to the formation of the family as a social institution. For example, Foucault (2003b) discusses how the family became instituted as a site of responsibility for the health of children as a consequence of the alliance between Christian discourses of the flesh and sexual psychopathologizing in the 19th century. More specifically, he argued that medicine somatised masturbation in ways that helped legitimate 'a new organisation, a new physics, of family space' (p.245). As well as opening up parent–child relationships to medical rationality and discipline, a part of the contract was that the family give the child up to the state for wider aspects of his or her education.

The duties of this new responsibility included intense surveillance over who had contact with the child's body and vigilance over the child's own relationship to its body, particularly while asleep. Only parents should be involved in the care of the child, no one else should have access to their body (servants, for example, should be excluded). And parents should be most watchful to prevent the child from becoming a masturbator, because masturbation was being considered as the root of most illnesses. Foucault suggests this combination of discourses helped deconstruct the extended family and constitute the cellular family as the key site that takes responsibility for the body and life of the child.

Surveillance over health and development also became instituted as technology through child health checks and clinics, especially after the Second World War, when primary health policy extended the medical gaze to the body of the growing child. In the UK this policy of surveillance was explicit and was instituted as a legal requirement. Within these child health screening and surveillance programmes, the bodies and behaviour of babies and children were compared with developmental norms. These were derived from the alignment of paediatric medicine and developmental psychology with population-based statistics.

As a site of biopolitics, discursive formation of the family focussed on the body of the child and this gave legitimation for the family and even the home to be entered and surveyed. This was the task of primary health care professionals, such as health visitors (Bloor and MacIntosh, 1990) who were charged with monitoring and measuring children's bodies and behaviour and holding these against norms of healthy growth and development (Purkis 2002, 2003). The effect was to further intensify the cellular nature of the family, as well as raising its significance as a site of care for children's health.

Alongside the intensification of the family as a cellular social unit and the institution of parenting as a site of children's health promotion, there is also the management of risk. For example, the US Environnment Agency (undated) directs parents over how they can protect their children's health, such as helping children to 'breathe easier':

- Don't smoke and don't let others smoke in your home or car.
- Keep your home as clean as possible. Dust, mold, certain household pests, second hand smoke, and pet dander can trigger asthma attacks and allergies.
- Limit outdoor activity on ozone alert days when air pollution is especially harmful.
- Walk, use bicycles, join or form carpools, and take public transportation.
- Limit motor vehicle idling.
- Avoid open burning.

Parents' concerns over the progress of their child are inevitably intensified through these discourses and programmes. So much so that parents' raised awareness can in turn be used to legitimate developmental surveillance as a clinical strategy, both in the UK, Europe and the US. However, it is not just child development and protection that becomes pathologized by these discursive practices, aberrations in development and growth are being tied to parental practices. So too diet and exercise, as well as methods of discipline, are read through observation and measurement of the child's body and behaviour. These measures inevitably become the cipher of good parenting, or evidence of abuse and neglect.

Parenting the 'healthy child'

As Armstrong (1995) notes, child surveillance renders both the physical and psychological growth of the child as inherently problematic. State surveillance of children is thought to have been much reduced in the UK over the past 20 years, with Bellam and Vijeratnam (2012) arguing there has been a shift from a screening to a health promotion discourse. This has meant greater emphasis on 'health education' and the institution of parents as having added responsibility for the identification of problems in their own children.

These discourses have helped to constitute the very notion of 'parenting' as taking proper responsibility for the health of the child in terms of stimulation, environment, diet and discipline. For example, Derbyshire (2012) examined research on the growth of children's brains that supposedly evidenced the consequences of not providing an enriched early learning environment in the first three years of life. Within this positioning, parenting is a part of the actor-network 'public health', in which the child is not only configured as at risk and in need of protection, but as also needing stimulation and enhancement in their environment.

The effect is disciplining, in that a particular view of parents as responsible for the health and development of children is reinforced. Consequently, parents are also being made *accountable* for their children's health and development in ways that go far beyond the mere protection of them from health hazards. Accountability for the normal, or even enhanced growth and devlopment of children is thus shifted onto parents: so that it is parents who are directly responsible for their child's development as well as their health (Lee 2001, 2009).

The medicalization of childhood and the family is thus producing a 'parenting culture' as a modern, political invention. This is something that is itself instituted. As Fairclough and Lee (2010) note, parenting is not only a social practice with profound existential as well as fiscal consequences, but has become an increasingly politicized site in which 'parenting' has 'acquired a particular place in contemporary society, in which the burden of managing risks is increasingly devolved onto individuals and families.' Mothers and fathers are continuously incited to be parents of a particularly moral kind, and in ways that take no account of social inequalities in people's means and capacities to be able to fulfil these kinds of moral elicitations (Skeggs 2010).

Most significantly for my argument, all this pressure to connect parenting practices with the physical development of the child (e.g. Kukla 2008) suggests that a realignment of the family and medicine might be taking place. For example, in pointing out that a core theme of contemporary UK social policy is based on the view that science leaves us with no uncertainty that 'poor parenting' is the main cause of social problems, Lee (2012) draws attention to the primacy being placed on the significance of 'nurture' and a commitment to recasting the relation between 'the family', 'parents' and the State as the key to a better society. That this view implies an intensification of medical research and technology – including perhaps being able to quantify the negative impact of neglect on the developing brain mentioned above – is something that has to be squared with the fact that provision of the 'right' kind of environment for a child to thrive is increasingly cast in terms of matters of consumer choice and the management of risk. I turn to this topic next.

Looking good, lifestyle and choice

The family is also being reinvented as a site of lifestyle, consumption and choice (Beck-Gershwein 2002; Smart 2004). The bodies and minds of children can be understood to be part of the on-going project in which consumer choice can be displayed and demonstrated to be effective. This is presumably more effective than the so-called 'Nanny State' in matters of managing children's health development.

In this scenario parents are not only to choose the best education for their child, but there is actually a global industry aimed at inciting parents to buy them a healthy lifestyle: food, clothes, gadgets, toys and so forth. There is an ever increasing discourse over which kind of activity, gadget, toy or food will or will not stimulate a child's development, help promote their health, and/or minimize their risk of harm.

At the same time there is growing emphasis on children's appearance: not just in terms of health and happiness but also in terms of looks and fashion. In contemporary life bodily aesthetics is connected to health through consumption: to look good is to look healthy (Featherstone 2001). Here parenting, and parent choice, is therefore also entangled in the fold of preoccupations with relations between health and bodily aesthetics.

Consequently, inasmuch as children looking good help parents to look good as *parents*, it is parents who are under surveillance – notably by other parents, as well as by government bodies. In addition for the children to be looking good means that they are also read as healthy and good. Yet things are never this simple.

It is not just that children's bodies can be monitored as a material semiotics that assists in the assessment of parenting. The *identities* of people, not just as parents but also as 'persons' and 'citizens', is entangled in how their children 'appear'. How their children look and behave, how healthy and happy they are, how well adjusted, how successful – all these markers conjoin as emblems of good parenting, and of their being a 'good' (morally, fashionably) person and member. Other researchers have noted some of this relationality between parental identities and how a child looks and behaves in the idea of courtesy stigma (Birenbaum 1992; Gray 2002; Green 2009; Goffman 1963).

For children to look good and healthy is also seen to be desirable because the idea of their 'looking good' helps display the parents' 'goodness'. What counts as goodness depends of course upon context, but people do feel open to being judged through how their children appear and particularly so in terms of how they look and behave. Not looking good, in both senses of the word, also throws the identity of the child into question. And of course children themselves, in assessing what they see others getting, also carry out much of this identity work on parents.

In summary of this section I am suggesting that children act as parents' 'extensions' in making their performances of identity and personhood (see also Hacking 1986). What I want to underline, though, is how parenting remains a moral, as well as an aesthetic, affair for parents. In reinforcing parents' positioning as responsible and accountable for the health of their child, keeping the children 'looking good' has today become a priority in parental identity work. I now go on to press how these associations connecting the family and health make up a complex site of identity work, one in which parenting remains enframed by a discourse of children's health, but where their performance of morality is increasingly entwined with consumption and choice.

Family and the medicalization of selection

So far it has been argued that the family is seen as the key site for the socialization of children as well as for the management of their health and development. Next, I discuss the degree to which family, in the context of a proliferation of genetic technologies, is also being installed as a site of selection. Rao (1996), for instance, suggests reproductive technologies 'do not simply transform the ways in which we create families. More fundamentally, they transform our very understanding of the term "family"' (p.2). In exploring how the new genetic technologies in my study affect understandings of family, I focus on families reproducing children deemed to be 'genetically' unhealthy or disabled. I should emphasize that in the clinic even a child (or their sibling) can, for a moment, be refigured as what I want to call a 'future parent', to legitimate the need to know more about their genetic makeup.

Parenting, in the context of reproduction, cannot be regarded as simply an extension of the actor-networks of public health promotion or reduced to the provision by families of a healthy lifestyle for their children. Rather there is the vexed question of new eugenic possibilities. Here, diversity of choice is expected to iron out cultural dominance in selection (Rothman 2004). This is because notions of desirability and perfection in children are themselves supposedly diverse (Condit 1999). Bauman (2003), in particular, links this last emphasis to the new consumerism – as the New Consumers, people have what he refers to as a 'bewitching prospect', a world of reproductive and genetic technoscience that will give them:

> [T]he chance to (and I quote Sigusch again) 'choose a child from a catalogue of attractive donors in much the same way as they [contemporary consumers] are accustomed to ordering from mail-order houses or through fashion journals' – and to acquire that child of one's own choice at the time of one's own choice. It would be contrary to the nature of a seasoned consumer not to wish to turn that corner.
>
> (p.40)

For this and other reasons, there is general disquiet among social philosophers over the wider and unintended effects of geneticization, particularly with regard to the emphasis on autonomy and choice (Egorova et al. 2006). For example, there are fears that discourse in genetic debate and policy over the use of genetic and reproductive technology promotes individualism in ways that risk marginalizing communitarian views (e.g. Habermas 2003; Parker 2000). Put bluntly, there are fears that the ways in which the new reproductive and genetic technologies are being made available will mean that some people will be able to 'go shopping' for babies (cf. Condit 1999; Human Genetics Commission 2004). What people will look for in children, as objects of consumer choice, are cultural notions of perfection (Condit 1999) or 'value for money' (Bauman 2003).

Contrastingly, Bauman goes on to observe that children are demanding in ways that also jar with 'value for money' as the basic ethic of liquid modernity. He suggests this is because children are dependent and constitute the kind of obligation 'that goes against the grain of liquid modern life politics and which most people ... zealously avoid in other manifestations of their lives' (p.41). For Bauman, then, offspring represent the stumbling blocks to liquid relations and to the rendering of children as mere objects of consumer choice. Children are the residual friction to too much emphasis on the ease of lifestyle, as matters of autonomy and freedom of choice. This, for Bauman, will save reproduction from the life politics of liquid modernity: children put a stop on what Bauman calls 'liquid love'.

However, in the light of issues discussed earlier in this chapter, Bauman's view does not take into account the jointing of morality and choice in relation to children's health. Specifically, 'soft' eugenics can be sanctioned as a process of selection in the reproduction of children diagnosed with genetic problems. Such sanctioning, as the analysis in previous chapters indicates, takes place in the context of understanding what appears to be rational, reasonable and moral given a particular family's specific circumstances.

Within this context there is certainly greater consensus over the need for selection as a matter of parental choice. However, as Stewart (2004) amongst others has shown, the very notion of choice is performed, not in relation to matters of 'consumer' choice and individual preference, but as an aspect of responsible parenting that promotes healthy children:

> DNA-based tests are now available for many rare genetic diseases caused by lesions in single genes, and couples who know they are at risk of having a child with one of these diseases can be offered an antenatal test to see if the foetus is affected. Sadly, no genetic disease can as yet be cured in the unborn baby – so the couple's only options if the test is positive are to terminate the pregnancy or to prepare for the birth of an affected child. The options for families faced with this situation were widened when the technique of pre-implantation genetic diagnosis (PGD) was developed in 1990. PGD involves producing embryos by 'in vitro' fertilisation using the couple's eggs and sperm, then removing a single cell from each embryo and testing its genetic material to see if the embryo is affected by the disease for which the family is at risk. Only unaffected embryos are used to establish a pregnancy. PGD, although it carries all the risks and stresses of IVF, nevertheless enables the couple to avoid the traumatic decision of whether to terminate an affected pregnancy. Previous surveys have shown that most people in the general public accept these uses of genetics to enable reproductive choice, provided the decision is made freely and without coercion by the couple concerned.
>
> (Stewart 2004)

As can be seen from this citation, there is general acceptance that those facing the reproduction of children with genetic problems should be given a choice, provided they choose in an environment free of coercion. So wherever the characteristics of children are medicalized and seen as pathological – for example, where a foetus or an embryo is judged to be affected by a gene disorder – parental choice over whether to dispose of some embryos or foetuses rather than others is sanctioned.

The consequence of all this emphasis on choice is that family becomes the site of selection, with parents being made accountable for their choices over the reproduction of potentially 'unhealthy' or 'disabled' children. This discourse over selection thus plays into and out of a very particular relationship between the family and medicine that relies on the medicalization of relations between parents and their children. So how does the relationship between parents and children become medicalized in the context of genetic medicine? As I show next, this process appears to rely heavily on the interaction of the clinic and the family.

Parenting and genetics

As I have discussed, the family has long been a social location instituted as a node in the actor-networks of public health, a site where mothers and fathers are instituted as doing parenting, and who can *choose* a lifestyle for their children to minimize risks and dangers as well as help promote their health and development. Alongside this positioning of family, parental identity work is entangled in how their choices reflect well on them. If these are the conditions of possibility, the historical complexity that prefigures interaction in the dysmorphology clinic, what do the various mothers and fathers become in the context of the genetic clinic?

We have already seen examples of the extent to which the dysmorphology clinic enters the family. Dysmorphology is grounded in the family as a social entity, beginning with early visits by specialist nurses (like Susan in Chapter 6) who survey the parental home and elicit information about the extended family as made up of both biological and social beings. We also saw how parents are involved in the construction of the family tree during this home visit, in ways that associate biological family and reproduction with the development and health of children, including how they look and conduct themselves. The information gleaned at the home visit is then carried back to the clinic. But the home visit can also be understood to do more than this – it paves the way to the family's attaching themselves to the clinic. In addition we saw how clinicians such as Professor Fox have to 'pass' with the family, as both expert and fellow human being, in order to further attach to the family as their extensions – their eyes and ears. But there is further complexity here.

At some moments, the family tree, in configuring the relationship between family, reproduction and the health and development of children, simply confounds the health promotion discourse with its emphasis on lifestyle choice. Specifically, in the genetics clinic, parents are not particularly figured as consumers who can simply choose a lifestyle to promote the health of their children. Rather, they are figured more as biological beings, whose bodies connect to other bodies as complex sites of reproduction. Here for example, is Kevin's father:

FATHER: Just thinking of anything else really about why, like I said, I have got such a big family and cousins you know, why didn't it happen to somebody else in the family, why me. You do think that. Me myself now, I've got four brothers and they have got big families, and why on my side? And the other thing is we've always been the fittest … before Kevin was born we had Tim obviously, we were always the fit family because we're always doing things, running, going on holidays abroad, everything sporty and then it happens to you, so you think 'why me'? *You know, it shouldn't happen to people like me because we've always had a lifestyle sort of busy and always doing things,*

no 'it's not going to happen to us', but it does happen, happens to everybody,
no matter how fit you think you are or you know, it happens to you.

(Emphasis added)

In Kevin's father's account we can hear that he knows what every parent knows: that he is himself under surveillance even while he is surveying others, in this case his brothers as parents. But we also hear more than this: the questioning, the disappointment and the bafflement. Kevin's father cannot understand *why him*? He was the very one amongst his brothers who most chose ways to live that would produce a 'fit' family. As far as he is concerned, he is the one who has been active in promoting a healthy lifestyle for his family. The logic is that, as a consequence of his choices, they should all be healthy. It also moves him to reassert his belonging – he is not just one of two parents, managing the lifestyle of his cellular family, he is one of many brothers, his children have cousins, and so on and so forth.

Under the conditions of possibility already discussed, Kevin's father made the right lifestyle choices; he has, in his view, been doing 'good parent'. As I noted earlier, in the usual relations between medicine and the family, the health and conduct of children's bodies are the material semiotics through which parents are judged. Under the usual deal through which parental identity is accomplished, he should have had healthy children: his children should look good on him. But he hasn't. Instead, he has got Kevin. His bewilderment expresses something else – that he feels that this is something out of his control.

Specifically, the clinic in dysmorphology makes people like Kevin's father very vulnerable because it takes some of the ground from under his feet as an agent: he is confronted by the view that making (good) lifestyle choices is not enough to make good children. Within his account we can hear how parents like him are exercised by both surveillance and a notion that they should be able to do and be good parents through the lifestyle choices they make. Yet we also hear that there is something about a genetic problem with a child that seems to confound autonomy and the power of choice. While the clinic in dysmorphology helps reinstitute parents as family members, it reminds them they are procreators, people who *make* families, and that procreation can be a precarious business.

Family matters in dysmorphology

As we have seen, geneticists' diagnostic practices, or categorical work, in dysmorphology constitute 'family' as a set of partially interconnected relations, one that may express a phenotype. The analysis earlier in the book noted how the child is a proband and documented how the referral of such a child to the genetic clinic is just the beginning of a process of investigating the family and building a family tree. The child thus acts for the clinic as a point of access to these family relations. So, as I have illustrated in previous chapters, the clinic grooms these relations in order to make visible what the laboratory cannot yet reveal: how to differentiate between occasions when some syndromes are the expression of a phenotype–genotype relation and times when they are not.

In this perspective of dysmorphology, family is far from being performed as the nuclear family of contemporary Euro-American social organization. Nor is it just the extended family constituted through a proliferation of *social* relations. Rather, family in the dysmorphology clinic is extended along the lines of biological relatedness, up, across and down the generations. While biological family members may or may not have been socially close previously (Strathern 1992c), the family tree and other aspects of diagnostic practice in dysmorphology open up the possibility that those who were socially 'far' become 'near' because they display parts in common. MacLaughlin and Clavering (2011) refer to this as the 'rekinning' that goes on in paediatric genetic clinical practice.

As such the family in the clinic is fabricated from the stuff of nature, but a nature that is organized through social and cultural associations – by marriage and so forth – not just by biology. It is these ideas that are made manifest in the image of a family tree or medical pedigree. So this way of enacting family brings the extended nature of family back into view.

Parents are re-instituted as mothers and fathers, brothers and sisters, daughters and sons. No longer just parents, they are reinstalled as *procreators*, as people who inherit the stuff of life from previous generations and pass this on when they make children, including those parts that are creating problems:

SALLY'S MOTHER: But you blame yourself, you know you blame yourselves, like we had done it, it's our fault she got this because it's genetic, that's what you've got to remember, it's genetic, it's come from the family, that's how I connected … genetic is followed down the family, we were trying to think who had anything wrong with them in the past. [Sally was diagnosed with *Cri du chat* syndrome, a new genetic mutation, soon after birth.]

But clinical processes in dysmorphology do more than face families with the possibility of defective genes. As I showed in Chapter 8, it makes some families stand for a syndrome–genotype–phenotype relation.

Poppy and her mother, for example, provisionally have become a portrait. A portrait not of a mother and child per se, but instead a portrait of the genotype that produces a phenotype, Kabuki syndrome. What such a portrait is suggesting is that somehow or another Kabuki is a family matter, in two senses of matter. The family has both something the matter with it, and the matter is to do with the substance the family is made up from: the matter that forms the basis of their living form. And here is the rub: such portraits emphasize that this substance is as much socially constituted as it is genetically composed. This is because these portraits record how family is made through social as well as biological associations.

Thus, in contrast to discourses of child health promotion, the bodies and conduct of living children – melded together with their distribution of signs across the family – are neither being scrutinized in dysmorphology to assess the parent's competence *as* parents, nor being judged over their capacity to choose a lifestyle and nurture a child into health and good citizenship.

In the genetic clinic the relationship between parenting, lifestyle choice and nurture is not viewed as greatly relevant. Even the diagnosis of the living child's troubles is only a small part of the story. In their place, as we hear in Sally's mother's and Kevin's father's accounts and as we have seen in how dysmorphologists work in previous chapters, there is an entry into the biological life of the extended family that reinforces a relation between the flow of matter up and down the family line on the one hand, and the health, shape and form of a child on the other.

In the dysmorphology clinic parents become engaged in a discourse that connects kinship and biological associations to the troubles their children display. As I have already evidenced, clinical surveillance of children's bodies is very much a part of both clinical *and* parental work – children's bodies are scrutinized as well as measured against particular statistic-based norms of child development and growth. However, the surveillance, as we have seen, also extends to other family members. Children's troubles are refigured less as the effects of lifestyle choice and nurture, and more as the effects of Nature – the hidden matter distributed across the family. So procreation, the bringing of people together into reproduction, is risky and needs, like everything else, to be managed through *counselling* people over the genetics of their reproductive relations.

Genetic counselling

The genetic clinic has explicit work to perform: the management of the reproduction of genetically problematic offspring. Thus the clinic is not only charged with diagnosis, but also with providing what clinicians and others refer to as 'non-directive genetic counselling'. Genetic counselling is represented as an event through which families become informed of the facts about their family and the risks of reproducing a child with a genetic problem. Genetic counselling is also represented by geneticists as non-directive – that is as concerned with providing information about 'what is', rather than involving itself in 'what ought to be'. It is a process which is informative and supportive but in which: 'Patients and their families are expected to formulate their own decisions, based on their personal, social and financial circumstances, and their religious convictions.' (http://www.usd.edu/med/som/genetics/curriculum/3CGENER3.htm) The difficulties of actually managing to fulfil the ethical standards of non-directive counselling in practice are well rehearsed by practitioners (e.g. Clarke 1991; Mahowald *et al.* 1998).

This work of counselling is not represented by clinicians in my study as 'curing the flesh' or as intervening directly in any disease processes – there are no surgical operations, transfusions or other treatment regimes offered in the dysmorphology clinic. Instead, the main thing offered to parents by the clinic in dysmorphology is *information*:

> Yes. And also I mean how we talk to patients … That's part of what they take away um, really. And part of their treatment really because we don't really

have, most of the time there's not a tablet or something you can do to change your genetic makeup. So what you can do is to allow people to have sufficient information and to inform their perception of what's going on.

(Author interview with Dr Barry, expert in dysmorphology, 2003–2004)

Many of the clinicians I spoke to emphasized the extremely delicate nature of this work of 'talking to patients' and of giving them information. This is because, they suggest, talking to parents is about making them aware that their child's troubles may be something genetic and that it may have been passed on. In their accounts this requires an intervention in how a family thinks of itself.

Clinicians enact this process as a matter of helping people like Kevin's father to 'think' *family*, not just parenting. In the clinic, this means getting him to think of himself and of his family not just as a place that nurtures and socializes children, or even as a biological entity. Rather it is a matter of getting parents and other relations to think of themselves as 'growing' progeny, as embodying the basic materials for growth; and that the substance the family is made up from may have a problem when it comes to the shape and form of the children that they make.

In order for this to happen, clinicians say that they have to go very slowly. In the following extract Dr Williams, a leading expert dysmorphologist and one of the recognized mothers of dysmorphology, describes these aspects of doing dysmorphology with the family as follows:

Aah, well, that's [sussing out what it is all about for the family] what you have to ask *them* [the family]. And this is what you have to start by ascertaining at the beginning of [the assessment of the family], you know, 'Who sent you? What are the questions? Who's asking them, is it you [the family] or is it the doctor?' You know? Who's got worries? Sometimes they say, 'Well I'm not worried but the doctor sent me.' Or, 'I don't know what it's about.'

(Author interview, 2003–2004)

Dr Williams is pointing to the intricacies of the consulting process and how she needs to assess the family in terms of how it already thinks of itself, including whether it has any inkling that there may be something wrong with its basic fabric.

She is suggesting that she needs to suss out its knowledge of itself and its motivation – what does it, the family want to know. She goes on to explain why:

But you've got to know there's other stuff uhm because that becomes awfully important in the way that you transmit the information back, because I look at it very much of, in genetics in general, I think of it [the family's situation] as a, uhm, a garden. And that you've got to assess your soil and your sunlight and your bits and pieces and your shadows and whatever, before you plant your information, and *occasionally* there's a hell of a lot a mess in that garden that has sometimes you just got to just clear *that* out before you even attempt to plant anything in at all; so I think of the communication and the consultation as planting information in a garden and you, for it to take or to, not to wither or to or to be constructive, or to be helpful, or not seen as another mess [laughs], you got to actually assess where you're putting it [laughs], at what time you're putting it, you know, and what, what else is going on because you're just one [laughs] little factor in these people's lives, which is enormously complicated, and so, you come in and you go out and you know, you, so your effect is, you know, can be unpredictable and so you got to think about what you're doing.

In Dr Williams' metaphor, families are partly natural – but they are not a wilderness; in her view family is more like a garden.

This is a complex idea because a garden is a form of (dis)organization (Munro 2003): a site where nature is enhanced by culture. And, like gardens, the organization of the family-garden can be problematic, disorganized and in need of cultivation: it can be overrun with weeds, just as the soil can also be poor. But weeds here are to do with both knowledge and the family's conception of itself, as well as the products of conception. 'Family' needs nurturing and tending in order for the strong plants to grow and the weeds to be quashed.

As such family is being performed here as a site of nature-culture, but one that needs an expert to manage it. It is being managed through changing its knowledge of itself. It is not that culture (scientific and medical knowledge, genetic medicine) can help improve on nature (the family garden) in any direct way. The consultant geneticist in this extract is not talking about genetic engineering. Rather, the genetics clinic is reinstituting the family as a social and biological group, and, as such, as a site of biosociality (Rabinow 1992).

The clinic is being refigured as a site not just where diagnoses are made but as where *information* about the family produced by the clinic can help the family to re-cultivate, and re-form, itself. To achieve this the family needs to change how it sees itself. Before the garden can be seeded with new information, the gardener needs to assess the light and the soil and clear the mess. The light and soil is the nature of the family, the mess is not just its deformity, but also the way that it sees itself. The implication is that its self-understanding is deformed and based on misinformation, and that it needs to be reformed through becoming informed. The deformation of the family is the effect of the syndrome itself on family members and relations, as well as the effect of misunderstandings and the family's incorrect knowledge of itself and its parts. The genetics clinic is as much about working on the mess and confusion of the family-garden to prepare it for reseeding as it is about reseeding the garden with new information.

Implicit to Dr Williams' discourse here is the idea that seeding information in the family garden will re-form the garden: by becoming in-formed (about itself) the family will then grow into the future in a different way to the de-formed way it has been growing in the past. This image of the family as possibly deformed and in need of transformation legitimates a process of *informed* choice making. Thus, when the clinic is in the mode of ordering that it calls genetic counselling, family is produced as both a site of reproduction and of biological relatedness as well as being like a garden; a nature-culture site, a space of biosociality made up of matter that need cultivating.

In this mode the clinic itself becomes a site of social transformation, while holding together two grounds between which it switches. Reformation of the family can only be accomplished through changing how the family-garden imagines itself, particularly in terms of its own biology and nature, its matter. And this change is to do with the family becoming in-formed. In this discourse, the clinician emerges not as embodying the scientific gaze, ready to answer questions on her or his work at the whiteboard of collegial discussion (saying what they see), but visualizes her or himself as the 'gardener', one that has the expertise and the know-how to bring about transformation of the family garden. In this way information is never neutral but is constituted as germane material through which the family tree can grow differently in the future.

Conclusion

In this chapter I have been at pains to elaborate how 'family' doubles for two conceptions of family: as a social institution hosting the lived relations people have with one another and as the carrier of biological matter of which a family is made up. It is a twin institution, holding together both that which is lived and living and the biological matter that is passed on through generations. In this doubling we can see how the biopolitical aspects of clinical work in dysmorphology extend from the behaviours and health of family members to their very fabric. This then is a site deeply engaged in the biopolitics of matter (Papadopoulos 2011).

As we saw in Chapter 8 on dysmorphology's portraits, family is produced as embodying the features or shape of a phenotype. To reiterate, by assembling and juxtaposing different images of 'affected' persons who are biologically related in the work of establishing the pathological, the genetic clinic is also enacting the relation between the syndrome, phenotype and an invisible genotype. Specifically, a phenotype distributed across different persons who are (assumed to be) biologically related to one another, is suggestive of a genotype that may run across a family. In addition, there are relations between the phenotype–genotype expressed across different generations of a family – as in the case of Poppy and her mother. These suggest the *possibility* that there are processes of inheritance at work here, but that the genotype is either passed on in an indirect way or in a direct way not yet fully understood.

In this perspective the family is transformed into a site of science, not in the sense of a laboratory experiment, but of a science observing the laboratory of life, one in which classification is still primary. The result of diagnosing (or not) abnormalities in children, is one of family being enacted as a potential site of science in which the relation between a genotype and a syndrome may be being produced and reproduced. Thus there is the question of risk, and of whether the abnormal phenotype or syndrome, and the particular formation of persons and their parts typical of a syndrome, can be passed on down the generations and through a family line. And this is something that the geneticists that I interviewed often mentioned: how genetic accidents can run in families to produce a phenotype–syndrome.

As I have clarified in this chapter, while dysmorphology overlaps with previous discourses of health promotion and earlier programmes of surveillance, it is not directly concerned with policing or assessing mothers' and fathers' parenting skills. Even when it rides genealogically on such discourse, we have seen in the case of Kevin's father how genetic possibilities bring the parenting culture up short – 'good' parenting alone won't help him in the face of a genetic problem.

Where families produce syndromes they are enrolled into the discourse of genetic counselling as possibly in need of *re-formation*. Assessment in the dysmorphology clinic here, though, is more about people's *procreative powers*, not in relation to their fertility but in relation to the *kinds* of babies they make and the kinds of babies that they might make in the future. Indeed assessment, as we heard from Dr Williams, is also about something even more than this: assessment is also of *family*, extensive families and family members, their social associations and reproductive powers. So at the same time as the clinic reinstitutes the family as a site of biosociality, it also harbours its access to the family, not just to parents. In the following chapter I show how transformation of the family is accomplished in its exchange of gifts with the clinic.

11 Transforming family

Having a baby has always been one of life's lotteries: boy or girl; dark or fair; large or small; will the child be free of inherited disorders, or affected by them; will the baby be completely healthy or will he or she have health problems? In recent decades this powerlessness in the face of chance and biology has begun to change.

(Human Genetics Commission 2006, p.4)

Introduction

I have begun to press how in genetic medicine the clinic is concerned with much more than either individuals or parents, or even, for that matter, treatment. Indeed we have begun to perceive how the family is reinstituted as much more than either a social institution or a site of parenting and lifestyle choice. Rather, genetic medicine helps reinvigorate the family, takes it beyond being a site of biosociality, and institutes it as the place where syndromes are produced and reproduced as entities, which require managing.

I ended the previous chapter with a discussion of how medicine's entry into the family is not only legitimated by the need to diagnose a child's troubles, but also by a 'moral' concern to investigate whether a family may need reformation in order that the reproduction of genetic disorders be managed. In this view, any member of the family (offspring, sibling, parent, cousin) who may be affected by an aberrant genotype becomes a 'future parent'. This has led me on to suggest how the clinic in dysmorphology is being installed as a site of biopolitics of identity, ontology and 'matter' (Papadopoulos 2011).

Some of the vulnerability of parenthood incited by the medical gaze in extension with genetics is captured in the above epigraph in which Baroness Helena Kennedy QC, Chair of the UK Human Genetics Commission, states that, as procreators, we are at the mercy of chance and biology, as though this were a matter of fact. This rendering of reproduction is, of course, not a matter of fact but is a discursive construction that invokes the matter of need: the need to think carefully about our decisions and our social and biological associations, including who we reproduce with, as well as who we reproduce.

Baroness Kennedy goes on to say that there is already technology and knowledge through which we might begin to manage this difficult state of affairs:

> Techniques of prenatal testing and imaging can now reveal if the unborn child has one of a number of serious disorders; parents can seek to terminate an affected pregnancy. Developments in genetic analysis and reproductive technology have now driven the point of decision making to the very origins of the embryo. Although still minimal in scale, limited in scope, and controversial in practice, some choices about the genetic make-up of our future offspring are already a reality.
>
> (Human Genetics Commission 2006)

Kennedy's rhetoric here emphasizes the enabling and empowering aspects of new technologies to reduce an impending calamity, and avoid being at the mercy of chance and biology. In this discourse, technology extends autonomy and decision-making to choices over the genetic makeup of our offspring, and even to 'the very origins of the embryo'. At the same time she is stressing the ethical profundity of such power. So, her discourse is set up in ways that install the need to regulate our decision-making and our choices.

As I have suggested in the previous chapter, regulating choice is partly a matter of instituting the family as a site of selection, and instituting the clinic as a site that oversees how decisions are made. In the UK this is the space of genetic counselling, a space in which selection over reproduction is legitimated through the pathologizing of particular kinds and forms of life. But what discourses over genetic counselling as a form of regulation do not illuminate is how genetic counselling, in the current context of clinical practice, is not a separate mode of ordering from the diagnostic process.

My point here is not that genetic clinicians set out to influence people's choices through transmission of their own values. It is more, as we have already witnessed in earlier chapters, that arriving at a definitive diagnosis in dysmorphology is far from straightforward. We have seen, for instance, the endless deferral over classification. We can also understand that this deferral links back to the root of the problem of establishing whether or not there is a need to exercise choice over reproduction.

In the context of what I have already shown about the genetic clinic in dysmorphology, the positivism inferred by discourses of genetic counselling rests on a notion that, as Baroness Kennedy puts it, there are tests that can reveal problems in unborn children and embryos. Yet this way of regulating reproductive choice masks the realities of how classification is accomplished on the ground. In addition, following Foucault (2003a), the positivism performed in discourses of genetic counselling is not simply hard to defend, but actually ignores how the need for choice is itself constructed.

In the chapter that follows I focus on how diagnosis as a protracted process of deferral engages families in very particular ways. Focussing on the interactions of family members and clinicians, I examine what is distinctive about these interactions. Specifically, what I illustrate is how parents in dysmorphology are not policed or disciplined in such ways as happens through the actor networks of public health. Nor are they simply excluded from diagnostic process. While my data suggests they are never simply 'informed', what the current study demonstrates is how families are gathered into the diagnostic and classificatory work of the clinic. In looking at this, I go on to explore how participation in the epistemological practices of the clinic has its own ontological effects, particularly where diagnosis is often elusive and where clinical practices are marked by explicit deferral and undecideability.

Performing good parent

In the dysmorphology clinic parents are not simply told the results of investigations, or just installed as witnesses. On the contrary there are complexities here, with some parents bringing the results of investigations with them. In fact, as we have already seen in earlier chapters, parents bring many things with them to the clinic: not just their child, but also sometimes their other children, as well as other family members, either literally or virtually, in the form of photographs and descriptions. These complexities are now discussed to illuminate the different ways in which the family is involved with the clinic and incorporated into its processes.

Parenting in the genetics clinic, as discussed in the previous chapter, is performed in ways that reinforce both traditional and contemporary notions of 'good parenting' (Daly 2004). On the one hand parents are enrolled in the clinic through the invocation of traditional cultural repertoires. By figuring children as 'becomings' (Lee 1998), interactions incorporate parents as the agents of society, working hard nurturing and protecting the young, controlling and disciplining them to aid their socialization, monitoring their progress and helping them to 'become' adults as normally as possible. On the other, in a more contemporary mode, parents are enlisted as experts – on their children: 'I always say to parents that you are the judge of quality of life if he gets ill. You are the experts' (Dr White to a parent).

This enlisting of parents might be thought to reflect the current emphasis in health care policy and practice of involving parents in the work of child health promotion discussed in the previous chapter, but there is more going on in the genetics clinic than this. In the dysmorphology clinic parents become fully engaged in the processes of objectification through which the abnormalities of their child's condition can come into view as of *clinical* significance.

The systems of distinction through which both abnormality and the genetic are evidenced engage the participation of the family in the *definition* of the problematic, and even the pathological. Specifically, to constitute something as abnormal, there have to be processes of comparison in play, systems of distinction by which comparisons can be made. Sometimes these are social, everyday systems of distinction. For example, a grandmother says of her grandson, Roger, that he 'runs like a poof [a homosexual]', thus drawing on a gendered discourse that distinguishes between how boys run from how girls run, and, further, that a boy that runs like a girl is like a homosexual.

This finding is important because earlier research on clinical contexts involving family members, particularly paediatric clinics (e.g. Derbyshire 1994; Purkis 2003) has emphasized how both patients and family members are excluded from participation in the definition of clinical problems. Specifically, these studies emphasize that the understandings and knowledge of parents and other family members are marginalized and excluded in relation to the clinical aspects of a condition.

Critically, as a social institution made up of differential relations of responsibility through which the pathological can be normalized (Foucault 2003b), family is reinforced through clinical work. In particular, David Silverman's (1987) studies of paediatric clinics show how the clinic is a site in which family as relations of responsibility is accomplished and policed. This said, while Silverman shows how parents and children alike are disciplined by clinicians' discourses to comply with medical orders, there is not the same degree of parental participation in the definition of *clinical problems* as there is in the dysmorphology clinic. It is this observation that prompts me to ask, first, how is this participation accomplished? And, second, what does it in turn accomplish?

In what follows I press how this participation in clinical process engages parents in exchanges of perspective on the dysmorphic child, exchanges through which possible (and sometimes implicit) explanations for their child's troubles come into view. Thus the child becomes, at moments, the complex and diverse object around which relations between parents and clinicians are accomplished.[1]

Encouraging participation

A practice that objectifies and reifies persons is nothing unusual and not necessarily diminishing (e.g. Fernandez 1986; Latimer 1999). What is interesting, however, is how, in their relations with the clinic in the current study, parents are encouraged to participate in systems of distinction grounded in domains of expertise and technoscientific discourses in the definition of their child's *clinical* problems. That is, in their relations with clinicians (performed around the epistemological practices through which the child as clinical object is constituted and known) parents are being mobilized in a very particular way.

For example, one mother says about her son that 'the only thing that wasn't delayed about him was his smile'. Another corrects the doctor to speak of her baby not as floppy, but as 'lacking tone'. The concepts of 'delay' and 'tone', and of measuring a child against norms of progress, are very much the staple practices of paediatric clinics, ones that parents sometimes resist as incongruent with their own perspective on their child's development (e.g. Purkis 2003). Yet the ways that some parents in the genetics clinic draw on these discourses indicates that they are engaged in the clinic as knowledgable and informed consumers of expert discourses. They are performing themselves *as* 'good parents', as the kind of people who know how to use experts in relation to the care of their child's body and health. As Skeggs and Wood (2008) have pointed out, knowing how and when to use expertise is all a part of ethical and respectable personhood and parenting. Just think of the range of reality TV shows (such as 'Supernanny') and magazines that perform this relationship.

What appears extraordinary against this background is that the genetic clinic specifically encourages, and indeed elicits, parental participation. Unlike in accounts of other medical contexts, parents' knowlegdeability does not appear to disturb clinicians at all. To the contrary, clinicians frequently engage in long discussions with parents about the significance of particular effects that draw in detail from scientific and other discourses. Sometimes they even adopt the expert methods of representation of a child's malformations provided by the parents themselves.

These exchanges are very unusual in medical contexts,[2] and indicate a shift in how medicine is relating to its client over the definition of clinical problems. For example, in the following extract Johnny's father had accessed an Internet site that graded scans of brain malformations (pachygyria[3]) from grades 1 to 5. Johnny is a toddler who has severe epilepsy, and severe physical and learning difficulties, including feeding problems. He requires total care. The consultant geneticist adopts the grading system provided by the parents to rate the child:

[Both Dr White (CG) and Johnny's father are standing at the light box examining the brain scans of children with severe pachygyria. The mother is slightly back from the group and very quiet, looking on, carrying Johnny on her hip. The scans are changed back to Johnny's scans and a scan of a normal brain.]

FATHER: These dark lines are too thick in effect [pointing at a scan of Johnny's brain].

DR WHITE: Yes, this is what the normal convolutions should look like [points to a normal scan] in the front. Johnny has poor gyri [the folds of the brain] but the cortex is not as thin as normally.

FATHER: So Johnny's brain is [like] none of these [pointing to the abnormal scans]?

DR WHITE: Yes, he is on the milder end. So Johnny has a pachygyria where the cortex is not as thick [as other worse cases of pachygyria].

FATHER: Which is good?

DR WHITE: Definitely milder, it only affects the front two thirds of the brain and spares the back of the brain.

FATHER: Is it possible to link the parts of the brain with function?

DR WHITE: You should be able to but it doesn't always work that way. The back of the brain in the integrated view (of Johnny's brain) doesn't seem to be affected, he is visually alert and inquisitive and a lot of learning depends on the connections they can make. There are a few things where it is understandable why he is milder, so generally this is a much milder scan than we would normally see.

FATHER: Good.

DR WHITE: It is also more unique. I've probably seen 6 to 7 children with more of a pattern like this [pointing to a very abnormal scan], [Johnny's scan] is more marked in front but grey matter is not that thick, so unique in the pachygria.

FATHER: In the US there is a grading system, 1 to 5, from the Internet. Based on what you said it sounds like a 4.5.

DR WHITE: I could do that, he's milder than that, 5B. Shall we sit down and I'll explain them? [They move into the other room.]

For a moment, at the light box, all Johnny's troubles are being given definition as the effects of his misshapen brain. Johnny's father performs himself at the screen as not just informed by systems of distinction and processes of comparison, but as learning to make readings of the scans by engaging in the epistemological practices of the clinic. Surprisingly, in a reversal of the usual interaction order of medically centred interactions, it is the father that asks the questions and makes comments on the clinician's judgements.

The scans reify Johnny's brain and enable his father to perform a detached view. At no moment does Johnny's father re-personify Johnny's brain scan. In contrast, the consultant shifts between moments in which the scans are reifying Johnny, and moments where he is re-personified ('*he* is visually alert and inquisitive', '*he* is milder than that'). So Johnny's father and the consultant talk about these parts of Johnny in a way that is cool, collected and politically correct: Johnny's father is folded into the clinic as, like the doctor, rational and detached. As evidence the scans are hard to move out of the way, but rather than just reducing Johnny to his scan, the doctor is issuing a more holistic, interpretative and inconclusive view of Johnny and his troubles.

In this way, the consultant's response to Johnny's father is inclusive as at the same as time it massages his perspective. It is reminiscent of the old adage that the most persuasive kinds of moves are those where the person to be convinced is allowed to think they thought of the idea first. The comparisons between normal and abnormal brain scans particularize and materialize Johnny's disorder: they make visible in material form 'what is' and what can be rated through processes of comparison. In so doing the application of statistical technologies brings into play the question of how extreme Johnny's disorder is. While his scan is milder than most cases that the consultant has seen, it is still very abnormal. But, and this is critical, it is not *normally abnormal*. Johnny's pachygyria (misshapen brain) is unique, and so is Johnny. Johnny's brain is at one moment being constituted as the same, and the next as different.

Inculcating motility

The call is for Johnny's father to be more than a good 'somatic citizen' (Rose and Novas 2005): that is, someone who has the will or desire to have knowledge about his child's troubles. The encounter between the consultant, the brain scans and Johnny's father, goes beyond grading Johnny's abnormality through processes of comparison. What is happening at the light box is a way of defining Johnny's troubles, and evidencing their severity, at the very same time as it holds Johnny's brain on ambiguous ground: it is neither completely fish, nor completely fowl (Douglas 1966). As an effect of this undecideability, Johnny's father is also caught in this space of motility, shifted back and forth by the consultant's shifts between definition and deferral: between processes of objectification and processes of personification, between material evidence of abnormality and processes of interpretation and judgement in which everything becomes tentative again.

When parents become engaged in surveying and assessing their child, they take part in processes for gauging their child's health and development. In this way they become enrolled in technologies that help visualize their child's health, including measures of assessment and practices of comparison. Thus, through the processes of 'becoming informed', parents are at moments moved by the clinic to help to hold specific aspects of their child against the technologies of a 'normalising judgement' (Foucault 2003a). In so doing they seem to be performing a different kind of parent to the one who is tired and up all night with a hyperactive child, or one who is attempting to encourage and support their child's socialization and development through practices of control and stimulation. These parents are consumers of expert and scientific discourses, willing and able to talk the talk of the clinic.

Yet in the specific moments in which they are being encouraged to engage in these discourses, they are also being exercised and moved by the epistemological practices of the clinic. As we have seen in the case of Johnny, these epistemologies may hold a child's diagnosis in a space of deferral, uncertainty and undecideability. Thus in being engaged in the processes through which they are becoming informed, parents are entangled in motility – the motility that shifts them between definition on the one hand, and undecideability and deferral on the other.

We should be careful here. This kind of motility is not to be conflated with Victor Turner's (1967) liminoid space of sequestration, the occupation of a space in between two status positions. While a space of motility heightens the parents' susceptibility to the exercise of power, it is accomplishing something different to the Ndembu rites of passage. Unlike the neophytes of the Ndembu, the parents are being moved about through participation, rather than sequestration and subjection.

Parents are shifted back and forth between a space of definition on the one hand, in which they are helping to see how their child's troubles can be known as belonging to a medical category, and a space of deferral on the other, in which the category is not yet fully known. The hinge between definition and deferral is the promise of a future of knowledge, provided the right path, the path that the parents have already experienced in the framing of what is already known, is followed. Whether to follow or not is of course left up to Johnny's parents. But what I want to emphasize, is how the framing of Johnny's troubles has prefigured this idea of choice.

Making it unique

As evidenced in earlier chapters, dysmorphologists spend a lot of time taking, examining and circulating photographs and slides and composing family histories and medical pedigrees. As already discussed, the photographs include family photographs with which they can compare family members.

Parents bring much of this material to the clinic and pass it on to clinicians. They provide photographs of the child over time, and of their siblings and other family members, and sometimes of themselves when they were younger or as children. We also saw in Chapter 6 how during the home visit parents give their accounts, histories and descriptions of other family members to the clinic. They continue to do this during the clinical sessions.

In these ways, parents pass accounts, photographs and other representations of family members to the clinicians. These representations of children and other family members become signifying clinical objects through processes of scrutiny and comparison. The use of slides and photographs helps reify aspects of family members through effacing their face as signifying personhood and identity (Bauman 1990, 1991; Goffman 1999). As effects, the photographs are not only treated as if they are immutable mobiles (Latour 1987), they help make people's most personal, social and human of parts (particularly the face) into things, the currency of the clinic.

Dysmorphologists enrol family, especially parents, not just in the work of supplying photographs, but also in the work of interpreting features and of distinguishing what is 'familial' from what is unique or syndromic. They elicit family participation in the practice of looking across family members for similarities and differences. This work of distinguishing things that are familial from things that might be 'just him' or 'just her' runs alongside the work of differentiating features and other aspects of children as signifying pathologies. If it's 'in the family', it may be an inherited condition or may just be familial; if it is not in the family, it may be a *de novo* event. For example, the extract that follows involves Patsy and her mother. Patsy is a 16-year-old girl with suspected Noonan syndrome:[4]

MOTHER: One thing I have mentioned to the other doctors, before I knew I was pregnant I was taking paracetamol and antihistamine.

DR LITTLE (CG): I think that is unrelated … I think it's a change that has occurred for the first time in Patsy.

MOTHER: I've got a couple of cousins and one has a couple of similarities.

DR LITTLE: What about Patsy's father's side?

MOTHER: He has a small family.

DR LITTLE: What's his height?

MOTHER: Normal.

DR LITTLE: It's possible Patsy might be the first person. [Turns to Patsy] You're unique; you're a special person, the first person to develop these problems.

Patsy's mother begins to enact a discourse of parenting that is caught in the mode of public health: that something to do with her actions has had effects on the child – in this case taking antihistamines and paracetamol while she was pregnant. But Dr Little disposes of this as irrelevant – the change has occurred in Patsy for the first time. Patsy's mother then passes more information to the doctor: that she has cousins who have similarities. Then in response to the doctor's questions about the father's side, Patsy's mother comments that his was a 'small family' – the doctor checks whether she means in height – the mother responds, no, height was normal.

Family members get enrolled in the work of ascertaining whether some of the things about the child that appear unusual or abnormal, such as their height, are clinically significant as signs by holding them against other family members. Features and parts of children in the clinic are thus compared with features and parts of parents, grandparents, siblings, cousins, aunts and uncles. Particular faces and facial features, including sizes and shapes, may not be abnormal, but 'in the family'. Other parents, like Patsy's mother, engage in this work of distinguishing the things about their children which are like other family members, but which may also be signs of a syndrome, particularly where they run through a male or female line.

As in Johnny's case, the consultant thinks Patsy is unique. Further, as with Johnny, it is the consultant who, however clumsily, re-personifies Patsy ('you're a special person'). Once again, we arrive at a moment where having been looking for what is the same, the clinician arrives at what is different, and in this case unique.

Is it in the family?

Importantly, clinicians involve parents in the work of tracing a feature or characteristic through the family, as well as in the work of differentiating the familial and connecting it to the work of identifying the pathological. In the following extract, the consultant is examining a young boy called Thomas while his mother is with him. They have already ascertained that Thomas has significant developmental and behavioural problems. Having taken a history, the consultant does a physical examination:

DR WHITE (CG): [She flexes Thomas's arms and asks him to squeeze her hands. She uses a tape measure to measure his head circumference. She feels his head, looks and feels his ear, looks at his face – one side and then the other side. With her finger she traces the space from his eyes to the top of his ears. She holds Thomas's head and looks at the back of it and leans over him to look at the top of his head and his forehead. She looks at his ears and the back of his ears. She then uses her stethoscope to listen to Thomas's chest.]

MOTHER: It's interesting mine's 52 [her head circumference], I'm on the lower end of the 'centile.

DR WHITE: We'll have to look at you later.

[Dr White looks at Thomas's feet and checks his reflexes. She notes a birthmark.]

MOTHER: Yes, I had one of those apparently.

[Dr White asks Thomas to stand and examines his feet. The nurse takes Thomas out of the room to measure his height.]

DR WHITE: Can I measure you? [Dr White measures the mother's head]

MOTHER: Yes, I have a small head.

DR WHITE: 53.3.

[Nurse and Thomas return]

[Dr White and mother check her head circumference on the charts.]

MOTHER: That [small head] could be the Polish genes [the mother's own father is Polish], unless that's what you get with syndromes.

Thomas's mother and the doctor together do the work of tracing a feature of the child (his small head) through the family and hold it against population-based technologies of normality (percentiles of head circumference). The mother herself suggests that the small head is in her family, and may be an expression of a 'Polish gene' rather than a syndrome.

At other times it may not be the size or shape of a body feature, but a medical condition or a particular characteristic or behaviour that parents help to trace through the family, both back through the line of the family and across generations:

FATHER (OF JOHNNY): He has a bit of eczema.

DR WHITE: Is it in the family?

FATHER: Not really.

Parents thus help do the work of comparison and are engaged in the construction of representations of the family that trace characteristics and pathologies across different generations or help ascertain where something about the child is different. From these tracings the clinic constructs the medical history of the family as well as a family tree. These technologies materialize, and therefore make present, the *possible* relation between developmental problems and other pathologies of the child's body, the family and reproduction. But they also highlight what does not yet fit, what needs to be known because it is different.

Is it in the genes?

I want to emphasize how parents and others bring the family to the clinic, so to speak, by passing on information, accounts and material representations of family members to clinicians. But it is also important to stress how clinicians either hold these things in play, or dispose of them as with things such as Patsy's mothers comment about taking drugs in pregnancy. In this way, medical discretion is operating in the clinic through parental participation in the clinical work of classification.

As I discussed in Chapter 3 the genes that are constituted as disordering bodies (and minds) are performed by the clinic as *not easily seen*. Clinicians cannot always send off blood or other samples of DNA for laboratories to look at to reveal the specific genetic pathology, although they are committed to a future of such certainty. Rather, as has been noted, clinical dysmorphology draws various clinic-based technologies together in the work of categorizing patients.

I have already shown in Chapter 8 how the gene type as the force behind the child's condition is made present through the alignment of multiple materials attesting to abnormality. The assembling and alignment of photographs and slides, test results, brain scans, medical pedigrees, family trees, and charts of growth and measurement not only helps make the abnormal visible, it positions the genetic as the origin of the abnormal, whether present or absent. Through these assemblages, which I have called dysmorphology's portraits, the genetic is given material extension as the ground of explanation for a child's troubles.

The accumulation of accounts and materials evidences (or not) the possible relation between the phenotype (features and medical histories traced across individuals and families) and the genotype. It is the very multiplicity of these materials, and the specific ways in which they are assembled and aligned, that supports the presence (or absence) of *the genetic*. In particular, even where a genetic diagnosis is not fixed, these assemblages magnify the possible *presence* of the genetic and attest to the probability of a genetic explanation, as opposed to some other explanation for the troubles a child displays.

The accumulation of this material evidence means that the genetic is made visible *over time* in other ways than, say, Johnny's brain is in the scan. Indeed, through these processes of alignment, the materials of extension feed off one another. So much so that the gene becomes enlarged, even huge. Meanwhile, other possible explanations for the aetiology of pathology are diminished.

As we are beginning to see, processes through which the genetic becomes visible rest upon the participation of family members – particularly for the construction of these materials as forms of evidence. Critically, for a genetic explanation to begin to take a hold on parents, the evidence has to exclude other possible grounds of explanation for a child's troubles. As we have already noted in the exchange between the consultant and Johnny's father, parents are being prepared for a lack of definition. Where this is so, they may need to rely on the clinician's judgement and a more holistic and interpretative form of knowledge. Let us return for a moment to the consultation with Johnny's parents.

Dr White has arrived at the moment when the doctor can introduce the idea that Johnny's troubles have a genetic base. She has engaged his parents in processes through which Johnny's abnormalities have been evidenced and the association between reproduction, family and these pathologies put into play. Then this exchange takes place:

FATHER: So definitely a gene?

DR WHITE: Yes.

FATHER: I was worried about radioactive radiation, I'm worried that may have damaged my genes.

DR WHITE: That's unlikely; sperm is produced all the time, if you had him straight after that [exposure to radiation] I'd be worried but less likely. My experience is environmental and infection problems don't really produce problems such as this. So we're left saying that most likely it is a genetic cause, which doesn't mean either of you carry this, it can just occur for the first time.

If that's the reason then recurrence would be low. If there was a DCX[5] change, we could look at you [mother] but he hasn't and there's no indication it is due to the DCX gene. If we had to classify, then I'd put him in 5B.

Dr White confirms that it is 'definitely a gene'. Johnny's father says he is worried that something he may have done (such as working with radioactive material) could have damaged his genes, and thereby Johnny's. So here Johnny's father demonstrates how he has incorporated a perspective: he incorporates a substance that is genetic, and which is mutable at the moment it is involved in reproduction. The doctor reassures him it is not anything in the environment that has affected the genetic material carried by his sperm, which went into making Johnny.

Dr White also asserts that things in the environment or infections do not 'really produce problems such as this'. She also states she thinks that neither he, nor Johnny's mother, carry the gene. At the moment that enough evidence for the genetic as a ground of explanation to hold has been assembled, and despite the absence of a definitive test, the doctor also draws on the negative DCX test result to support the view that the problem is not inherited. So now the issue of any risk of a recurrence arrives quite naturally, namely that, because the condition is not inherited, the 'recurrence would be low'.

In the way the exchange develops it appears that the father wants certainty ('so definitely a gene?'), while the consultant shifts between a space of categorical definition (there's no change in the DCX gene) and deferral – *if* that's the reason, *if* we need to classify. Thus the consultant exercises the parents on the grounds of deferral at the same time as a genetic explanation for Johnny's troubles is able to exclude other possible explanations. So that the choice they see is from the perspectives that they are given. They do not choose of their own accord: they only see choice from the perspective given by one of the frames – definition or deferral.

The space of definition gives an essentialist framing, 'look here it is, this is what it is, it's genetic'. And the framing provided by the space of deferral constitutes these as matters *yet to be known*, and promises categorical definition in the future. Parents are not choosing these frames, but are instead being moved from one space to the other at, for most practical purposes, the discretion of the clinician.

A moment of arrival

Following this phase of the consultation, Johnny's father goes on to ask about prognosis. Dr White suggests that Johnny's case is 'milder than most', and that he will reach adulthood:

FATHER: The horrible question, we know it's not good.
DR WHITE: It's very individual, the information is very old and gives general survival rates. He's milder and a lot of these problems are feeding problems, and aspiration and epilepsy treatment has improved. Seeing him today,

there's no reason why he shouldn't grow to adulthood, but the overall lifespan is reduced. He's a very healthy young man and there's no reason for him not to grow into adulthood.

The presence of death is made explicit in the clinical assessment of Johnny's troubles. Johnny is re-personified – he is strong and healthy, he should live but only into adulthood, not beyond. The presence of the gene rules out other explanations for Johnny's troubles – his premature death and terrible troubles (epilepsy, delay, learning difficulties) are genetic in origin.

This motility between definition and deferral excites consciousness of danger and risk. The need to calculate risk over future acts of procreation is legitimated. Jonny's father is moved, from being a parent to becoming a 'future parent'. And, as such, it becomes imperative for the father to ask the next question, although Dr White has already slipped issues of recurrence into her assessment in the previous sequence. In doing so Johnny's father gives an account, an account that momentarily and temporarily disposes of any future children that might reproduce Johnny, not a reified Johnny, but Johnny as the child who is dependent and demanding:

FATHER: … Also a question was 'What's the risk of recurrence?'
DR WHITE: Unfortunately, the children I know don't have siblings. I don't know, about 6 [a 6% chance]. He [Johnny] doesn't have any other problems. DCX is normal, the gene is normal. I'll ask a research group in Italy I work with to look into this. Then we are left with the uncertainty, this is a unique situation, I may need to check if there were any other siblings.
FATHER: Of course we'd like to [have another baby], but for obvious reasons we don't want another Johnny, he's a lot of work.
DR WHITE: You're still young.
FATHER: I took drugs [amphetamines and marijuana] when I was young …
DR WHITE: Don't worry, I've not seen any association. It's genetic but not necessarily familial.

Dr White offers a calculation – a 6% chance of recurrence. In the clinic and in the family, only some genotypes are represented as *inherited*, others are identified as particular to individual persons, as spontaneous genetic anomalies. But when it comes to the risk of recurrence, families and future children can be constituted as susceptible to such spontaneous effects even if the risk is low. To be more certain regarding the risk of reproducing Johnny, the doctor will need to ask other experts.

In these ways the need for calculation, running alongside deferral, legitimates the need for more research, more investigation, more science, and more knowledge. But what for a moment gets disposed of is Johnny, or at least the spectres of Johnny reproduced into the future. Johnny is 'a lot of work' so 'we don't want another'. And to make things just a bit more sure, the father makes another confession – he's taken drugs. But he is reassured and absolved; it really isn't anything he's done – it's genetic, but it's not familial.

It is the practices of the clinic, and the constitution of the abnormal as matters of fact, that legitimate disposing of a reproduction of Johnny: by making Johnny's troubles the effect of his nature (his genotype), it becomes possible to dispose of him, figuratively, as 'a lot of work'. But critically, Johnny's father is now in a perspective, a perspective that at one moment enables definition and the next takes it away. The perspective troubles his conscience and moves him between his consciousness of his past and his future acts of procreation.

Ways of representing genes are not value free – only some codes and their expression are identified and categorized as 'normal', others are considered anomalies. The normality invested in some phenotypes and genotypes, rather than others, makes visible the kinds of characteristics of persons that are being valued, at any one time or place. Thus the ways in which genes and their effects are imagined, and classified, make visible the grammar of cultural codes of normality.

Significantly, it is the genes that are made pathological in the clinic: nature and substance are made aberrant, not persons. And it is the genes that are medicalized. In addition, it is Johnny's father, not the consultant that gives utterance to the disposability of a reproduction, not of himself but of Johnny. Johnny, through processes of objectification, has been detached – the reductive version of Johnny flows not from his father but from an aberration in nature. Johnny's father's detachment, and his shift in perspective, is facilitated by his engagement in the clinical processes of definition and objectification.

The need for a decision over whether or not to reproduce is thus passed back to Johnny's father, but only after it is enframed through the interaction in which Johnny's troubles are both medicalized and geneticized. While the ambivalence and uncertainty of cases like Johnny's can only be calculated and probabilities suggested, what is nonetheless being put into play is the view that a stop on the reproduction of a genotype like Johnny's is desirable and necessary. Although the doctor appears to retain her ethical delicacy as non-directive, she is at the same time managing reproduction. She is turning ambiguity into a resource (cf. Munro 1995) with which to manage the risk of reproducing people with long-term, chronic conditions like Johnny's.

The exchange of perspectives

In the clinics studied this is how genetic counselling is carried out. These different ways of representing genes and their effects interact *in use* with lived relations between people, primarily in the ways in which relations between persons are imagined (for example, in ideas of inheritance). But they also interact with the ways in which relations are *ordered*; for example, in terms of notions of responsibility for those characteristics of children considered anomalies.

We can see something of this trend in the next excerpt when we turn to Roger's mother again:

MOTHER: I was so relieved when I got your letter [saying that her son's condition has nothing to do with her kidney disease during pregnancy]. I blamed myself all these years.

DR SMITH: We can completely rule that [an event in pregnancy] out ... there's some type of genetic problem likely to have occurred with him, there's nothing running through your family, we've looked for fragile X and chromosomes.

In being given an explanation for Roger's troubles, that they are genetic in origin, Roger's mother is momentarily absolved of responsibility for them. It is nothing she has done: her identity as good parent, like that of Johnny's father, can be affirmed.

Yet, even at the moment of definition and absolution accomplished through the exclusion of other possible grounds for Roger's troubles, the tone of deferral is held in play, 'there's *some type* of genetic problem *likely* to have occurred'. This is one aspect of the exchange: Roger's mother brings Roger, and representations of other members of the family to the genetic clinic, and in return what she gets back is a sense of relief, a moment of exoneration of responsibility. Like Johnny's father, she is for a moment being affirmed as a good parent.

In my earlier discussion of the work of Marilyn Strathern, I noted how the child is the object of clinicians' and parents' relations of exchange. Questions arise therefore as to what it is that is actually being exchanged? I want to go on now to press that what are being exchanged are *perspectives*.

Participation in the construction of re-presentations of family substance creates perspective and reframes past and future acts of reproduction as potentially pathological. At the same time, the space of deferral excites the need for repro-ductive calculation and for more knowledge and more technology. Choice is framed and the need for 'information' elicited and prefigured. Parents receive a path of knowledge to follow, a perspective from which to 'see' things more clearly, now or in the future. This may well include intensification or exoneration of their own responsibility for their child's troubles.

Where the disordering of the genes is not being constituted as directly inher-ited, moments of reflexivity are incited through the ways that the genetics clinic materializes the *potential* relation between pathologies, death, family and acts of procreation:

MOTHER: I just thought Ross and I coming together had done something terribly wrong. I felt perhaps I'd done something wrong, with genetics I felt my child could die ... I'm not a medical person so I'm very ignorant but I felt a bit like cerebral palsy, something like that you know, or the sort of genetic prob-lems that I'd encountered were turning up [...] so they weren't nice instances, you know, it wasn't a case of something wrong but you can lead a normal life, they were 'This is going to be hard for my child'. [No diagnosis at time of study.]

This blaming of oneself is repeated by parents across the study. In these particu-lars, medical genetics offers some comfort to parents but, as we see next, this is not always so.

The exchange of hope

At the same time as scientific methods of categorization gives them a detached perspective that helps give a sense of order to the potentially unbearable, participation in the dysmorphology clinic also offers parents hope. This emphasis on the disturbance of self, instantiated by engagement in the genetics clinic, both overlaps and contrasts with Cussins (1996, 1998) and Moreira (2004). Moreira, for instance, demonstrates how patient participation in the socio-technical organization of medical work both calls for and mediates the 're-establishment' of self, including processes of detachment. In contrast, I am arguing that as parents become detached from one set of materials, they are attached to another. It is these shifts that change perspective.

What I turn to now is that the possibility of a genetic diagnosis may at moments take something away from parents, and even lead to 'all the hope' being killed off. The death of hope is expressed by Sally's mother in the following extract. Sally is a teenage girl with a diagnosis of Brachio-oto-renal syndrome:[6]

SALLY'S MOTHER: But to be told that it wouldn't be made better took all the hope away. To know it wouldn't get better. When we were told that it was not likely to be made better by Dr Jones when we first came here [to University Hospital] it was a shock. And all the hope was taken away. We were both in tears.

As this brief interchange makes clear, perspective is not set apart from the theatre of action, a 'being outside'. Rather there is a shift, back and forth, between spaces that grant perspective, and which enframe a view of the situation.

As we have seen in the analysis of the interaction with Johnny's father, the gift of participating in the clinic is a space of motility that offers a path to knowledge. This affect is expressed in the following extract in which Sally and her mother are talking about their experience of the dysmorphology clinic in an interview:

SALLY'S MOTHER: They [the geneticists] did tests. Well, the scans had already been done, so Dr Page [the consultant geneticist] looked at those and put it together. Because of the hearing and the holes and it fitted the criteria I suppose.

SALLY: And she looked at my hands and I had to do things like this [bends fingers] and she looked at the shape of my face. I think it was to see if it all fitted.

MOTHER: Yes, she looked at both of us, didn't she?

SALLY: Yes, and we didn't have the characteristics. And she took photos, too, to see [if] it fitted in with other people who have it.

MOTHER: Yes. I'd forgotten about that. Yes, she was very thorough.

INTERVIEWER: It sounds like you were looking for a diagnosis or [were] unaware of this for a long time. How did you feel when they referred you to genetics?

MOTHER: We were very pleased. Because we had nothing in Muddletown, and suddenly here they wanted to get to the bottom of it too. Before, I was a fussy mother who wanted to get to the bottom of it, but Dr Page did too. It was so good to have people doing stuff at last.

Sally's mother and Sally describe themselves as being transformed in the dysmorphology clinic: from people who have no idea why they are like they are, into people whose bodies are the objects of interest because they may represent something, something to get to the bottom of – an 'it'.

In this way, the clinic entangles people like Sally and her mother in an exchange of gifts (Strathern 1988; Sykes 2005). Parts of their bodies are objectified – 'she looked at my hands', the 'shape of my face', the scans – and 'she was very thorough'. They describe how they are in the gaze of the clinician, and their appreciation of the care that is taken. The doctor also tells them that they don't have the characteristics, but takes photos, to see if they fit with others. In turn, they feel that the encounter is full of promise: 'a way' that enables them to 'put it together', 'get to the bottom of it', 'see if it fits in', 'have people do stuff at last'.

'Unless you do research you can't find out'

The gifts the family pass to clinicians include access to the family and their genetic material, and consent to use these materials in future research. In return there is the promise of what Delvecchio Good (2001) calls 'medical imaginaries':

> [People] invest in the medical imaginary – the many-possibility enterprise – culturally and emotionally, as well as financially. Enthusiasm for medicine's possibilities arises not necessarily from the material products with therapeutic efficacy but through the production of ideas, with potential although not yet proven therapeutic efficacy. (p.397)

The gifts the clinic pass to the family are of a future, a future of definition, a future of classification. Hope.

That family members are being enrolled as *allies* in the making of these futures becomes at moments quite explicit. Here, for example, is another extract from the interaction in the clinic with Roger's family:

DR WHITE: I'm interested in movements. Roger was really good up there [on the examination table]. I'm interested in movements because a new gene has been identified, these boys have learning difficulties and some funny movements ... we're setting up this test in University Town and we could add Roger if you would like to go down that route ... that's the only idea I have at the moment ... I may have others in the future.

ROGER'S GRANDMOTHER: *Unless you do research you can't find out.* (Emphasis added)

This excerpt exemplifies the gifts being exchanged. The clinician will get to test Roger's DNA, and he will become a part of her research study on the genetic makeup of boys with funny movements and learning difficulties – boys like Roger. The grandmother gets the gift of participation in a medical imaginary and a future of defining the genetic unknown, and of eventual classification and definition that this future promises.

I am therefore suggesting that parents are moved by the materiality and the motility of the clinic in ways that construct particular moments of reflexivity. Parents become not just informed, but *transformed*. Transformation is accomplished not so much through the transfer of information, but through interaction with discourses and technologies that exercise consciousness and shift perspective.

At the same time as the clinic gives family members perspective (perspective on a way to knowledge, to definition and a future in which the disordered can be ordered and classified), the clinic gets the family enrolled into giving them the material they need to research – the opportunity to ground the relation between the genetic, dysmorphias and the pathological.

Definition and deferral

It is the child that becomes, in the genetics clinic, the boundary object (Bowker and Star 2000; Star 1989; Star and Griesemer 1989) that facilitates access and communication between the world of the family and the world of genetic science. Recalling Foucault's (1994) analysis of the two moods of science, as, on the one hand, being called to seeing 'the same' (the closed, that which is already fixed and categorized), and, on the other, to understanding 'the different' (the open, that which is still to be known and named), I want to suggest that participation in clinical work reinforces contemporary ideas of parenthood, including entangling parents in the ontology of a way to knowledge.

The space of definition – diagnosis – shows parents where things are the same. It emphasizes that categorization is possible, that medical knowledge practices have already been able to 'fix' things and are able to show 'what is'. This is, of course, an essentializing space. Contrastingly, the space of deferral reminds parents of the need for a path to knowledge that can deal with what is not the same, with what for the moment seems different. The space of deferral identifies the different, and promises that that which does not yet fit will be known. It will be fitted in and categorized, providing, of course, that the right way to knowledge is followed. The motility of the clinic between decision and deferral helps to hold (some) parents in the hope of a future of definition, and so entangles them further in the ontology of scientific understanding.

Doctors in the clinics I observed are thus managing reproductive choice, and the risk of the reproduction of children with potential chronic conditions, not through direct intervention but rather by drawing on ambiguity as a resource. The work of identifying the causes of troubles (as genetic in origin, or not, as inherited, or not) is marked by definition, undecideability and deferral. Therefore, participation in the specific epistemological practices of the genetic clinic moves parents between definition and deferral to entangle them in a 'space of motility'. Immersion in this space of motility, however intermittent and relatively brief, excites consciousness of the riskiness of reproduction, elicits moments of reflexivity and shifts in perspective through which the very need to 'make informed choices' comes into view.

As such, perspectives that are not of the parents' own choosing frame choices. So that as at the same time as participation in the clinic tasks mothers and fathers with choices through which the future can be determined, the clinic also entangles them in deferral, and the need for more knowledge, more genetic technoscience *and* more clinical judgement. The choice is to follow the path of clinical understanding, so that what is identified as different can be – if the well-honed path to clinical knowledge is followed – categorized as the same; as something that fits, something that can and will be categorized.

I suggest that the practices through which the clinic enrols parents and other family members in the re-representations of a child's troubles is a process of intervention *in its own right* that accomplishes shifts in parental, not clinical, perspectives. As Dr Williams in Chapter 9 puts it, the clinic works on the family like a gardener works on a garden with the tools of very specific and interactive communication practices and medical technologies to cultivate it and reform it. But the way of reformation is something the parents have to do themselves once their view of things is reframed. The outcome, as Dr Williams asserts, can be unpredictable: it is the unpredictability of persons, left to choose, that is accountable for poor decisions in the future, not genetic counselling. As other research has shown, what people do with what they get from the clinic is translated through their lives in ways that may differ from those intended by geneticists (e.g. D'Agincourt-Canning 2001; Konrad 2005).

Keeping the non-genetic in play

In raising these issues I do not want to be misunderstood as simply showing how practices of genetic counselling are socially constructed and socially constructing. Rather, I am suggesting participation in the epistemological work of the clinic raises the possibility that genes can have the kinds of effects that parents are seeing in their children. It makes the genetic as a ground of explanation for particular effects *present*, intermittently and temporarily, but still potently. At the same time this perspective helps exonerate parents from blame.

I am underlining, therefore, how genetic counselling practices can be understood as intervening, not just because they 'shift perspective', but instead because they *give* parents perspective. Indeed, they give them a perspective that moves them between two interrelated places from which to 'see': definition and deferral. This is not to suggest that what we have seen in the clinic is simply a process of geneticization – it is not a totalizing effect. On the contrary, many things in the clinic are not considered 'genetic'. In addition parents are encouraged in their nurturing and managing of the child to believe that biology is not all, that nurture and care have their place. But critically, rather than practices of representing being only concerned with a way of legitimating forms of intervention (Hacking 1983), representing in the genetics clinic *is* intervening.

Genetic medicine, then, is a critical site through which the genetic, as a domain of classification, is being embedded through the social fabric, at the same time as it is a site in which choice is prefigured and elicited by the motility of clinical knowledge practices. Choice in the genetics clinic is not performed as a matter of individual preference. Rather, in the genetics clinic reproductive choice is worked alongside the construction of risk, risks of abnormalities as the expression of aberrant genes.

As we have seen, rather than ideas about what constitutes goodness, well-being or normality being left to cultural diversity, in the clinic choice is prefigured through processes of objectification and the practices of the clinic that institute conceptions of abnormality as matters of fact. The clinic exercises parents as reproductive choice makers, but as choice makers whose choices are constructed not (or so it seems at first glance) by cultural expectations regarding normality and goodness, but by rational processes of objectification through which the abnormal can be defined and the causes of abnormality detected.

But of course clinicians are not representing themselves as doing that, as representing – they perform their assessment of the child and the family as a process grounded in the application of tools which allow them to reveal 'what is'. They perform their gaze as scientific. They make their way of representing the child's body objective through the application of statistical and other technologies. It is through the ways that parents themselves are engaged and moved by the epistemic practices of the clinic that they are moved, in-formed and their identity as calculating reproducers elicited.

Specifically, the genetics clinic brings death, disabilities and acts of procreation in relation to one another, thus confronting parents with a profound and shocking portrait of the latent potency of their own and their child's materiality. So, rather than these findings merely being evidence of a process of geneticization of medicine, and of the family, I want to stress how the alignment of clinical judgement, genetic science and the family gives greater opportunities for differentiation, not less, affirming the need for more discretion, reflexivity and calculation, not less.

In summary, the clinic certainly puts into play ways of conceptualizing ourselves as already incorporating the genetic as something 'that is'. Yet, through entangling parents in a space of motility, it also excites the need to know (more) about the embodied self in relation to science in order for us (and this may eventually be all of us) to make (good) reproductive choices.

Conclusion

There are two problems with the emphasis on autonomy and choice in current discourse over the use of genetic technology in relation to reproduction. First, as discussed in Chapter 10, recent research suggests consensus over the need for processes of selection where pregnancies risk reproducing children with severe disabilities, providing there is the science and technology to support informed and autonomous parental choice. As other commentators (e.g. Roeher Institute 2002) point out, this makes people with aberrant genes, such as Johnny, Roger and Patsy, readily disposable, and warrants a form of social exclusion. However, as Konrad (2005) has already shown, the conditions framing parents' reproductive choices extend far beyond the boundaries of the clinic, so that practices of inclusion and exclusion are emergent upon a complex ethics that is also local, relational and specific.

The second problem concerns the way that a relation between being 'informed' is put into play alongside the stress on autonomy and freedom of choice. This emphasis de-socializes 'decision', and decouples information as merely a means to select ends: as if choices can be informed and yet remain autonomous. This is not just to press the point, as others have done, that reproductive choices can hardly be taken in a social and cultural vacuum (Human Genetics Commission 2004). Rather it is to press the need to understand better how becoming 'better informed' involves processes that are never just means to ends, but are always to some extent (obliquely, indirectly and partially) constitutive.

The analysis presented in much of the book has demonstrated how the alignment of genetic science and the clinic gives medicine particular access to the family. It reinforces and plays upon contemporary conceptions of family as a site of *parenting*, a site that takes responsibility for the body and life of the child (Foucault 2003b). But it also does more than this.

Specifically, the clinic becomes a site of 'gathering' for the family, made up of both biological as well as social relations. Here family is being constituted as more than cellular: at least for the purposes of genetic assessment, the family gets re-extended. The notion of good parenting also becomes extended to include becoming responsible as 'future parents', both over how and with whom people reproduce and over how and by whom families are made. As we have documented, becoming 'informed' engages the participation of mothers and fathers, stepparents and grandparents, in the work of defining children's troubles – and by extension, possibly their own. And yet, for all that reproductive choices are emergent upon these processes of definition that redistribute family across many parts, the moment of reproductive choice still reconstitutes the cellular family as a site of parenting.

What gets black-boxed in professional and policy debate is how the very process of 'becoming informed' is not value neutral: it gives *particular* perspectives. Practitioners and policy makers may constitute clinical knowledge practices of diagnosis in genetics as simply revealing the facts of the matter. But in so doing, they reproduce medical theories that constitute the medical gaze as simply detecting and describing 'what is'. The problem with this view is that it effaces how medical knowledge practices are constitutive in themselves, only recognizing the effects of diagnosis if it is poorly executed or (however unintentionally) mixed up with moral agendas. This view of genetic counselling practices has already been critiqued as ignoring how clinical processes in genetic counselling construct the potentially affected future child as the abnormal Other (e.g. Roeher Institute 2002).

For the purposes of the present chapter, I have been pressing a different problematic. The analysis of parental participation in the genetic clinic offered so far has shown how the effects of parental participation go further than eliciting their performance as good parents, or even as good 'biological citizens' (Rose and Novas 2005). Indeed, I have shown that participation in the definition of clinical problems in the genetics clinic gives parents perspective in ways that have particular and important effects. Specifically, parents' engagement in the epistemological practices of the clinic entangles them in a space of motility that moves them to become more conscious of the riskiness of their own and others' reproductive powers.

The ways in which parents and other family members are enrolled in the representational practices of the clinic is itself a process of intervention through which reproductive choices are framed, prefigured and elicited. That is, participation in the epistemological practices of the genetic clinic 'moves' parents in particular ways. Specifically, through clinicians' shifts between moments of definition and moments of deferral, parents are held in a 'space of motility'. The space of motility excites a sense of reproductive risk and elicits moments of reflexivity to institute mothers and fathers as calculating reproducers, tasked with choices as if these can determine the future.

These findings show how the processes through which the need for calculation in reproductive decisions is elicited, in turn, helps to constitute a particular kind of personhood, a contemporary Western personhood. As at the same time as these Western persons are being made aware of the riskiness of their reproductive powers, they are also being figured as having the capacity to choose the future; but, and this is the point being mandated and pressed upon all of us, choices can only be responsibly made where the future is rendered knowable through the alignment of technoscientific innovation and clinical expertise.

At the same time, by shifting family members back and forth between the experience of definition and the experience of deferral, the clinic also constitutes parents as persons whose current choices cannot fully determine the future because 'more always needs to be known': in the absence of definition of what currently appears to be 'different', choices are being left to the vagaries of speculation and guesswork in the name of calculation and prediction. Parental immersion in the space of motility thus enrols them not just in the need for expert judgement, but in the need for more genetic technoscience. A technoscience that is yet to come, but one that will – through following the path to knowledge already presumed to be effective in the definition of problems – render the unknown knowable.

While I am noting how this participation exercises a new form of consciousness of people's own biosociality, including the riskiness of reproduction, I have also illustrated how families become the allies of the clinic. This is achieved through relations of exchange. Specifically, in their passing on information as well as bodies, accounts and histories of family members to clinicians, the family help the clinic become a site of gathering that reinstates it as the centre of discretion over the identification of need and the classification of genetic syndromes. In return, the family are given perspective on their disabled children, including exoneration of responsibility, and participation in a way to knowledge that promises classification of their troubles in the future.

Part V
Conclusions

12 Summary and discussion

The gene, hunted, inspected, tamed, or in the process of being tamed, participates in the construction of long and highly differentiated sociotechnical networks, transforming monsters into human beings in their own right, well integrated into constantly evolving webs of relations.

(Callon and Rabeharisoa 2008, p.40)

Introduction

A central argument in this book has been to show how an association with the gene is reinvigorating medicine. In looking at medicine's association with the gene I have also demonstrated that we are seeing a rebirth of the clinic, whereby the natural histories of 'syndromes' are being written in the clinic's immersion in the world of families. I carefully documented how this classification work in dysmorphology is helping to identify and differentiate certain syndromes as genotype–phenotype relations. I then illustrated how the clinic acts as a site of crossing between the 'grammar and codes' of molecular science and the 'living flesh and substance' of the phenotype. These findings led me to consider how the repercussions of thinking of family as partial expressions of a phenotype become embedded into the wider fabric of society.

In investigating this resurgence of clinical interest in congenital abnormalities, I widened the study to focus as much on the clinic's links with family as with its associations to the biological sciences. Here I have attended to what is termed 'identity work' in sociology and given particular emphasis to how clinicians must 'pass' with the family, one moment as 'expert' and the next as 'fellow human'. In return family members must 'pass' as worthwhile sites of scientific investigation, although the work they do in passing on family insights and stories to the clinic acts as a necessary but not sufficient condition for their inclusion. Over and above these exchanges, the clinic retains the authority to weed out what is unusual but not pathological.

In examining these complex relations between the clinic and the family, I have evidenced how the clinic constructs itself, carefully and cleverly, as a space of gathering into which the family are enrolled to 'gift' self-descriptions, photographs and histories, as well as material representations of themselves in the form of blood and other body products. In exchange for their involvement in the clinic, I traced how the family gain a 'perspective' that promises a future understanding of what is wrong with their child. Hope is deferred to a future of more research that will bring greater knowledge of themselves and their family.

Critically, and significantly, I noted how this engagement with the clinic includes family members experiencing switches in ground. Discourse in the clinic moves between methods of diagnosis that individualize at one moment to focus on the 'proband' – the child with troubles – and 'assemblages' that re-institute wider social relations in the next – as partial representations of a poorly defined and hard to see genotype. At the same time as the latter perspective appears to exonerate them of agentic responsibility for the condition of the present child, discussion over future reproduction faces them with the possibility that their genes may be 'out of control'. So simultaneous to the clinic helping parents to see that their offspring are not simply a matter of managing their lifestyle better, parents are nonetheless inculcated with the view that they may need to manage their future procreative activities to ensure that they do not reproduce another child with aberrant genes.

Dysmorphology produces and reproduces its powers of authority in all this through building and enacting a way to knowledge – an expert gaze – that is routed through a social and cultural assessment of family life, as well as involving assiduous clinical attention to the shape, form and function of its members. At the same time as this clinical gaze engages in procedures of refutation and cross-checking through the assembling of evidence, it sets up processes of differentiation which continuously press the possibility of doubt and uncertainty. Through these processes of deferral, the clinic greatly enhances its powers of discretion to differentiate between 'natural curiosities' and what is a sign of pathology.

It is this deep immersion in the family together with its enactment of the scientific method of doubt that re-accomplishes medicine as the site that can both 'see' and 'say' syndromes while differentiating their causes. And it is through this work of differentiation that the clinic re-enacts itself as a site of classification, although its work today is not so much the traditional role of separating the 'sick' from the 'malingering' but one of identifying those who may be genetically aberrant from others who are not.

What caught my interest though was the work of deferral in which probands whose diagnosis is uncertain were retained in the clinic. This last finding suggested that pivotal to the clinic maintaining its status as a science (and in rebuttal to views that would position it as the mere handmaiden of experimental science) is the way clinicians deploy this possibility of doubt and so balance decision with deferral in their consultations. This argument rests on two initial premises: first, and here I was drawing on the seminal work of Foucault on modes of science, that medicine is most dominant at the point where *classification* is central to its mores; and second, if less contentiously, that the clinic is at its most scientific when explicitly deploying the method of doubt.

The implication, although the point may already be obvious to many readers, is that science is only science when it is still 'in the making'. The genetic is thus for medicine a new frontier that is powering a resurgence of medical dominance because it reinstalls the clinic as the location of discovery. What is of particular interest in all this is that discovery here is not a matter of technologies or interventions, but of *understandings* about how humans are formed and grow. The discoveries of the genetic clinic concern garnering knowledge of how offspring are deformed and focus on when these deformations constitute things that are clinically problematic, not just in terms of individuals but also of families.

Additionally, and related to the on-going struggle for dominance between the medical and biological sciences, this close reading of how these two forms – classification and deferral – are worked together has also led me to conclude from the study that retention of the mode of deferral is as essential to the exercise of power as is the mode of decision. People may come to the clinic for diagnosis in the first place but they are only enrolled *as material for scientific investigation* where there is also room for deferral. I return to these matters below.

The theme of medicalization

What is compelling about the clinic is how it grounds its way to knowledge about the growth and form of persons within the actual relations of reproduction: the family and the mess of bio-sociality. This led me on to see that an end biopolitical result is how normal family reproduction is being medicalized through attention to the *abnormal*. As I have pressed, the normal is shrinking in the genetics clinic, so that the need to distinguish how, when and in what combinations, reproductive material may produce a syndrome is more and more engrossing – not simply to those families who have already reproduced what seems to be faulty but indeed to all and sundry.

Heightened forms of medicalization have interesting ramifications in terms of responsibility, but my point is not only with how the clinic augments its powers to exonerate or rationalize practices of exclusion. Rather the concern is over cultural preoccupations and mores, particularly to what 'fear and fascination with the deviant may lead' (Dikötter 1998, p.1). As Dikötter's study of Chinese policy over reproduction illuminates, the urge to draw clear boundaries between the normal and the abnormal combine with medical discourse to form 'a program of eugenics', including:

> 'the implementation of premarital medical checkups' to ensure that neither partner has any hereditary, venereal, reproductive, or mental disorders, the ordinance implies that those deemed 'unsuitable for reproduction' should undergo sterilization or abortion or remain celibate in order to prevent 'inferior births'.

> (p.1)

For all that genetic inheritance may be incomplete as grounds of explanation for human variation and complex human traits as a science, Kaplan (2000) helps us see how these kinds of explanations for human problems (and difference) not only helps construct the problems but denies other fields of explanation for their origin (p.184).

Contrastingly, what we have seen in the current study is that the clinic – especially in its mode of ordering referred to as genetic counselling – precisely acts to engage parents in clinical work, including uncertainty and undecideability over the classification of some troubles. In line with the neo-liberal way of contemporary biopolitical life, rather than the State legislating who should or should not reproduce, it is parents and what I am calling 'future parents' that the clinic involves as people who need knowledge. This is because it only installs them as decision-makers once their perspective has been framed through their participation in the motility of the clinic as a space of decision and deferral.

In pointing to these trends I am not at all proposing that the association of the gene and the clinic reinvigorates medical dominance for its own sake. Rather my thesis is that the historical place of the clinic as a social institution is being reborn in genetic medicine, and this draws on earlier contentions that medicine is the queen of the human rather than the life sciences. This isn't just because medicine, as my discussion of Rabinow in Chapter 1 suggests, is likely to be the key site through which the new genetics becomes embedded in society. Certainly I am suggesting that the clinic is the 'obligatory passage' through which the gene participates in the construction of the long and highly differentiated socio-technical networks referred to by Callon and Rabeharisoa in the citation at the opening of this chapter. But I am also suggesting that the clinic reinstates itself as a site for the protection of the human, because it shows how it is the syndromes that are the 'monsters', *not* human beings. At the same time the clinic, to its credit, sees those who collaborate and shelter within it as human beings of a very particular kind; that they have consciousness and are agentic and in need of knowledge. Genetic medicine in the clinic gets reinstalled as necessary because its combination of classification and deferral allow it to *moderate* how the genetic is embedded in society.

As I argued in Chapter 2, the clinic is historically a space of dividing practices between the needy and the legitimate and the rest. It is only medicine that has the authority to legitimate when to interfere in reproduction and when not to interfere on the basis of clinically defined problems rather than personal values. Thus it is the clinic in its association with the gene that, acting on behalf of society, starts to be instituted as a site to regulate the potential tsunami of genetic technologies. This is not so much, as I have shown in Chapters 9 and 10 that medicine overtly directs people with regard to their reproductive decisions. Rather medicine reasserts its ability to account for selection on the basis of need, rather than say consumption and desire. In this way medicine is also being reinvigorated as a social institution because its dividing practices, between the genetically problematic and other beings, acts as an indirect form of arbitration that mediates some of the excesses feared and foretold by the marriage of new genetic technologies and a culture of enhancement.

This biopolitical dimension of the clinic can be seen in how it works the family not only as a site for the production of syndromes, or reproduction as a site of potential risk, but to legitimate *selection* as a new dimension of contemporary parental responsibilities. Parents are not just to choose a healthy lifestyle to ensure the future of their family's health, they are also shown a way to produce the progeny that will ensure that future, provided they follow a specific way to knowledge – that offered by clinical discretion in the identification and classification of reproductive problems.

Drawing on my fieldwork I illustrated how doctors may do the work of categorization in different ways, but my analysis underlines how medicine continues to accomplish this classification work on persons *in the realm of the clinic*. This puts differentiation and classification, rather than therapies and interventions, as central to medicine's power.

The key concern for medicine is not its dividing practices, separating the sick from the deviant, or the normal from the abnormal (although in many ways it is here that medicine operates as a centre of discretion and so gains much of its power), but with performing itself as scientific. As Robert Nye (2003) has recently argued:

> Aiding and abetting the state in the growth of carceral regimes that segregated the deviant or marginal seems to have been far less important a motive than that of adding to scientific knowledge and practice that would redound to individual practitioners and to the independence and status of medicine as a whole (Bleker, 1997; Lawrence, 1996; Loudon, 1986). Scientific medicine, it would appear, and the continued rise in medical educational standards, was very much a product of the competitive dynamics of the profession, the ambitions and realism of young doctors, and of efforts to enhance the prestige, if not yet the efficacy, of the medical profession (McClelland, 1997; Solomon-Bayet, 1986).
>
> (p.122)

In making these points I acknowledge that I am writing in the face of the many social science arguments that point to how medicine's dominance is on the wane; and on the wane because of the erosion of medical discretion and the demise of the clinic. In what follows I therefore revisit these arguments before offering a theory of medical power that helps us understand how medicine continuously reinvigorates its dominance.

Rethinking medical dominance

As discussed early in the book, the thesis of medical dominance has long been a key debate in medical sociology. Its recent extension into Science, Technology and Society (STS) is linked to the proliferation of molecular and genomic technoscience and has led not only to ideas that medicine will be totally geneticized but also the theme that the clinic will be deposed. In Chapter 2 I began to suggest how medical dominance is partly achieved through medicine's alignments with other bodies and discourses in networks of associations and I now expand on this theme in the rest of the book.

In Chapter 3 we saw how in the association of the clinic and genetic science, bioscience is being ordered and reordered. Investment in more knowledge about the gene is being legitimated when it is demonstrable that more research is needed. Increasingly, however, the need for more research is demonstrable only if it can be shown how it will improve health or help the fight against chronic diseases in the West. This is partly an effect of the entanglement of Ethical, Legal and Social Implications (ELSI) of science and functionalist programmes that call on the biosciences to be more relevant and address society's problems and 'health needs'. But it is also happening because it is thought that it is medicine that adds values to science in ways that make it of value to society, including its translation into capital. Interestingly, then, what we are seeing in this deflection from 'bio' towards 'life' sciences is a medicalization of *bioscience*.

Potently, since bioscience has to show government and other funding bodies how it addresses medical problems in order to give it moral as well as economic purpose, I am suggesting that what may actually be happening in these alignments and shifts is an intensification of medical authority and discretion. The effect of such an intensification of medical authority can be seen, for example, not only in how 'access' and the entry into the domain of health care have become such crucial foci of health and social care organization and practice, but also with the intensification of medicine as 'gatekeepers' to the distribution of social goods, such as beds, investigations, medicines and care (Hillman *et al.* 2010; White *et al.* 2012).

In Chapter 4 I began to show how and when it is the clinic where the identification of the pathological occurs, not just the description of what counts as abnormal. My argument here is that, instead of witnessing a diffusion model of discovery moving from the laboratory to the clinic, what is witnessed in the classification of genetic problems is rather that it is the clinic that is enacted as the key site for the identification and description of abnormalities in the growth and form of human organisms. So it is the clinic that acts as a 'centre of discretion' over the making of *genetic* clinical categories; and it does so in ways that are infrastructural to new scientific enterprise and not just to health services.

In making this argument I identified several problems with how medical dominance has been thought of, and which I think has misled people into thinking that medicine's power is on the wane. First, there never was a 'golden age' of science and medicine as pure, discrete spaces for the production of knowledge about the natural world. It is not just that science and medicine have always been entangled politically, economically, as well as philosophically, socially and culturally, it is the attempt to split medicine from science that is a problem. In saying this I do not want to stress the social construction of scientific knowledge, but focus more on how any separation of medical and scientific domains is an *effect*. An *effect* that in turn is constitutive of culture, and a particular politics of the body, of persons and of families.

Second, in many debates about the relation between bioscience and medicine, science is conflated with the laboratory, while medicine is associated with the clinic. As I have suggested there is an intricate entanglement between medicine and science through which the clinic does not just use laboratory science but itself becomes a part of the scientific endeavour. In making this point I should stress that I do not mean an experimental scientific endeavour, so much as an engagement in the reading of nature concerned with the identification of problems, that is pathologies, that need to be solved.

Third, innovation and discovery are often more visible in science than in the clinic, because what we see in everyday clinical practice is usually what is already sedimented repetitively into routines. Typically classification is naturalized even though, as both Mol (2002) and Atkinson (1995) separately help to recover, diagnostic classification in the clinic is itself an effect of practices and processes of debate, negotiation and adjudication between different forms of evidence.

Fourth, there is a problem with dividing medicine and science into separate domains and then conceptualizing the flows of knowledge, discovery and innovation as just running one way. As has been discussed in Chapter 3 the diffusion model has many problems, not the least of which is that it underestimates the extent to which the emergence of biology and the molecular is also a history of the intensification of medicalization.

Fifth, there are questions over what are the 'commons' between bioscience and medicine, for example in terms of their sharing metaphysics, politics and ethics, not to mention the production, consumption and disposal of cultural preoccupations, values and mores, including ways of imagining relations themselves (Strathern 2009). When it comes to commons, the ground that bioscience and medicine share is not only connected to underlying notions of seeing/saying and assumptions that accredited ways of knowing can take us to the truth, to positive knowledge. There are also deeply embedded Euro-Western notions of progress lying in the realm of our will to 'master' nature, conceptions here including our own internal nature as well as nature external to us (Clarke *et al.* 2003).

As Fuller (2007) puts it in his consideration of how science maintains its dominant position in society:

> On both the technical and the ideological front, science's power as a form of knowledge has rested on its ability to justify practices that might otherwise appear illegitimate. This speaks to the transformative character of science ... even of the human condition.
>
> (pp.2–3)

In reflecting on the profundity of this thought, we might go beyond just acknowledging a need to remember how both medicine and science are material practices, or recognize how the jointing of the market and metaphysical values capitalize technoscientific domains (re-emerging perhaps as 'Biomedical Technoservice Complex, Inc.' Clarke *et al.* 2003; Rose 2007b).

Spaces of ontic politics

What I would stress more than the topical themes of material and capital, important as these are, is that science and medicine are also sites of ethical and metaphysical battles, or, to use Verran's (2011) term, spaces of 'ontic politics'. In this respect I have pressed how it is the *categorical* work of medicine, and how it not only defines what counts as need, but rather how it commits categories on persons – in the form of diagnosis by 'othering' them – that is key to understanding medicine's power.

There is though something particularly subtle in what I am addressing under the rubric of ontic politics that goes beyond traditional thinking about social exclusion. What has fascinated me in the present study is how medicine deploys its categories to include things and persons in one moment and uses them to 'other' these things or persons in the next. Much of the newer categorical work has been linked to the emerging relation between technoscience and medicine and commentators stress how new and emergent identities and subjectivities (Finkler 2000) are being fabricated. To give just a few examples: carriers (Attard 2009; Parsons *et al.* 2003), pre-symptomatic patients (Konrad 2005), prepatients (Rose 2007b) and biological citizens (Novas and Rose 2000), as well as new kinds of social formations (Callon and Rabeharisoa 2003; Rabeharisoa and Callon 2004; Rose 2007b) and new kinds of body-persons that imply different kinds of possibilities for ontology and biopolitics (Dillon and Reid 2001; Kelly 2006; Latimer 2013; Papadopoulos 2011; Rabinow and Rose 2006).

Critical investigation I feel is especially important over the relation between bioscience and medicine and its legitimation of innovations and new technologies as matters of need and expediency. Here we should try to interrogate how it is that the effects of bioscience and medicine in their alignment always go beyond the functionalities they promise – the prevention and cure of disease or the optimization and enhancement of bodies to promote health. The point here is to learn to see how they rather help produce, consume and dispose of particular meanings and moralities, as well as persons. In this I am bringing the politics of imagination (Latimer and Skeggs 2011) alongside biopolitics to understand how medicine continuously extends its power.

In arguing these positions I am purposefully extending Foucault's basic contribution to identify a way of thinking about how medicine extends its power. Following Strathern's (1991) lead I should say that I accomplish this in my fieldwork primarily through noticing processes of attachment and detachment. I look for the folding and unfolding of bodies. And I watch for the pulling and pushing of persons into and out of medicine's reach. Significantly, as I have illustrated in many of the chapters, the reach of medicine is extended in genetic medicine: from the locating of disease in the genes, and individual bodies, to the family: as I have noted many times, it is when a phenotype is visible across the bodies of family members that the genetic aspects of syndromes can be evidenced.

In this way I never see medicine as simply one thing rather than another. Rather it is bio one moment and social the next. Here we can understand that medicine's power and potential dominance comes from its shifts in extension, and not from its purity, except that as we have seen medicine still performs diagnosis as a moment of clinical purity. Critically, we need to understand more how medicine shifts between its hybrid associations to moments of clinical purity.

So rather than go with views that talk about the molecularization, and colonization, of medicine and the birth of a subjugated technoscientific medicine, I want to suggest that capitalization, technoscience and the new molecular biology have already been offering opportunities for medicine *to extend* and perhaps even intensify its power. Indeed, as I suggested in Chapter 3, the reverse may be happening in the medicalization of science.

To be sure, this requires thinking about contemporary medicine, and science, as well as their historical relations, differently from much current opinion. And perhaps in ways that I have been evidencing throughout the book, giving greater recognition to the view that medicine's detachments are as potent as its attachments, including, as I have also documented, those exclusions and inclusions that are so momentary that, in the next minute, they are gone. So I want to go on now to offer a different view on medical power and suggest a dimension to understanding medical dominance that has the possibility of problematizing Rose's and others claims. This approach may also help us to understand better how the genetic, like the car before it (Latimer and Munro 2006), is not just engrossing science and medicine, but the social body.

Towards an alternative theory of medical dominance

Setting aside arguments for the demise of the gaze and the flourishing of technoscientific medicine, I have been examining occasions when medicine 'does' something and carefully noted when it displaces its gaze to other technologies. Keating and Cambrosio's (2003) thesis of medical platforms, discussed in Chapter 4, in the constitution of medical entities is useful, but they do not engage with how alignments are accomplished on the ground. The question that needs to be asked instead is how, and when, does medicine attach to technology? And how, and when, do technologies magnify or diminish medical authority? Throughout this book, for example, I have been asking when does medicine do bodies as information and when does it do fleshy bodies as illness and disease?

Medicine's momentary attachment to and from technologies and others' materials and discourses help magnify medicine in ways that maintain rather than diminish its authority (Latimer 2004). For example, people can now pay directly for myriad scans, or online tests of their DNA, and they can acquire endless amounts of knowledge and information about their bodies and their health. At one level this availability of technology appears to bypass the need for doctors to order the tests. But can the results really be made to matter, for example in an insurance claim? Or legitimate absence at work? Or do they not usually require for their fiscal authority the sanction of clinical interpretation and opinion? That is, medicine's authority may appear displaced at some moments, but its intermittent exercise at key moments, and across key social processes, helps substantiate its orderings and stabilize its power.

Stability and social order can be understood, as in actor-network theory, as a process of aligning interests. As noted in Chapter 3 this is often thought to take place in 'the process that is called translation which generates ordering effects such as devices, agents, institutions, or organizations' (Law 1992, p.366). However, contra actor-network's notion of alignment as having to be stable to produce its effects, my argument is that alignment is often partial rather than total, or consistent. Indeed, the more partial the alignment, the greater opportunities there are for medicine to make switches in ground. In this perspective intermittency and multiplicity offer more, not less, opportunities to generate power effects (Munro 1995).

Specifically, what is missing from much research is a way to bring together notions of complexity (including the possibilities of multiple sites of medicine and possibilities for interpretation and conduct in the clinic) alongside this different perspective on power. Silverman (1987) captures some elements of this perspective in his conception of how a discourse of the social *extends* medicine's power. In my earlier work I tended towards showing how medicine's power and authority is extended, at particular moments rather than others, by its attachment to and translation of other disciplines and domains, including managerial technologies such as collaborative care, triage, multidisciplinarity (Hillman *et al.* 2010; Latimer 2004; White *et al.* 2012).

In this book I have chosen to emphasize how it is first in its moment-to-moment shifts between extensions (including deploying the gaze itself on occasions as a technology), and second in its enactment of deferral, that helps medicine maintain its power. My argument is that we need to attend to translation in the emergence of the genetic in terms other than a simple takeover of medicine by science and technology. We need much richer analyses of when and how science and technology extends and magnifies medical power and when and how it curtails and diminishes it. Here there needs to be analysis of how, and at what moments, medicine attaches to technologies and discourses, and when it detaches. In Chapters 9, 10 and 11 we saw how the clinical work of dysmorphologists helps exclude other grounds of explanation, such as lifestyle or environmental factors for a child's or a family's troubles.

We should also ask at what moments do clinicians attach to a scientific mode of operation, and when do they do something else? Similarly when does medicine perform certainty and positive knowledge and when does it do uncertainty and doubt (Seale *et al.* 2001; Star 1989). Further, when does it do fixed, managed medicine and when does it do the unknown? When does it do specialization and when does it do generalist? When does it medicalize and when does it de-medicalize? And critically, what gets accomplished at these moments of attachment and detachment, extension and diminishment? And especially who or what benefits (*cui buono*)?

Diagnosing dysmorphology

In the light of these remarks I now take the opportunity to review my findings noting that, throughout the book, medicine has been treated as a site of biopolitics as well as a social institution. What I want to summarize is how tracking the various and complex relations between the clinic, the gene and the family in dysmorphology has helped unpick ways in which medicine is reinvigorated as a site for the production not just the consumption of knowledge.

As we saw in Chapters 4 and 5 dysmorphologists figure themselves as discovering and establishing what they call 'syndromes' and this work includes passing the discipline on to neophytes. While in some cases the genetic basis of the more common syndromes can be 'seen' through the application of special tests, for many syndromes there are no tests. As such the genetic basis of a syndrome remains provisional, but is implicated by the assembling and interpretation of clinical evidence. Considerable stress was put by clinicians on the visual aspects of expert recognition, as well as their methods for making syndromes 'visible' by establishing patterns of signs and symptoms across bodily systems and across family members.

In Chapters 6, 7 and 8 we saw how dysmorphology makes use of genetic technoscience, some of the time at least. Surprisingly, however, methods of genetic profiling include many clinic-based technologies (such as the compilation of medical pedigrees, photographs and family trees) as well as laboratory-based methods of analysis. Specifically, clinical evidence of the genetic is generated through the various technologies enrolled in the clinic, including the gaze (Foucault 2003a) of the dysmorphologists themselves as well as their methods of genetic profiling. Collectively these technologies *materialize* what is abnormal or unusual about a child, as well as make a relation between these specific features and pathologies and the possibility of a genetic basis. In this perspective the disorderings of the child's body (and perhaps those of other family members), taken together, become a phenotype. As such they are being constituted as an expression of an aberrant, if invisible, genotype.

This possibility of clinical representation of a phenotype–genotype relation is partly instituted through dysmorphology's portraits. In my examination of dysmorphology's portraits in Chapter 8, I showed how the genetic clinic emerges as a space in which the relation between genes (codes and information) and living, fleshy bodies is given form. While 'morph' (from the Greek) denotes shape, it is worth us remembering that morphology is not just a branch of biology that deals with living forms; it is also a branch of grammar that deals with the formation and inflection of words. The two disciplines seem worlds apart, like the study of living forms, and the 'post-genomic' representations of genes as information, codes and rules. Yet in a sense what dysmorphology's portraits do is bring these worlds – the flesh and the grammar – into a relation because they help see/say a genotype–syndrome relation. Specifically, the ways in which dysmorphology makes its portraits creates a space of crossing, through which form is given to information (the aberrant genes) such that the gene is made visible and the gene is not just given presence, but is, for a moment, magnified.

I should take a moment to stress the kind of scientific work being enacted here: the method of assemblage and juxtaposition discussed in Chapter 8 is a mode suited to a correlational science looking to take forward *classification*, rather than it is compatible to an experimental science seeking causes. What I suggest these clinical methods of portraiture both reflect and constitute is the shift in genetic science from one gene as responsible for one disease, to the complexity of classifying a syndrome–phenotype as the expression of a genotype. Thus, the portrait is a way of representing syndromes that does not reduce them either to a single gene or to the figure of an individual and, instead, allows syndromes to emerge in the partial connection between the assemblage and juxtaposition of materials deriving from different, biologically related bodies. In this we can see how the clinic really is doing the '*new* genetics'.

These findings suggested to me that the models and textual discourse of the molecular and the gene mimic or simulate digital machines in ways that perform a different texture to fleshy bodies. As such the molecular gene brings with it a different, incompatible world to that occupied by fleshy, living bodies: these two worlds seem irreducible, they are in a *non-relation*, much as Foucault helps us to see the extraordinary space that is constructed through the non-relation between words (titles) and pictures (paintings) in his exposition of Renee Magritte's '*This is not a pipe*' (Foucault 1983). The implication is that the relation between the new genetics and strategies for the governing of life is *qualitatively* different from being the very long chain of translation that Rabinow and Rose (2006) think links the molecular and the molar – between information codes and the fleshy vitality of the individual human organism.

What we have seen is something more than this. There is not simply a shift from the molecular to the molar, from 'becomings' to the individual and the figure of enlightenment thought. It is not simply that medicine cuts down the solid figure of the individual in their differentiation of the molecular and the molar described by Deleuze and Guattarri (1987):

> There is no becoming-man because man is the molar entity par excellence, whereas becomings are molecular ... Man constitutes the majority, or rather the standard on which the majority is based: white, male, adult, 'rational', etc., in short, the average European, the subject of enunciation.
>
> (p.292)

What I have evidenced instead is how dysmorphology moves from clinical pictures of representative subjects to portraits of genotype–phenotype relations. This is a move, yes, from the molecular to the molar; but then it goes on beyond the individual to the *distributed* nature of genetic substance. So that the central thrust of biopower in genetics is in this movement because it radically extends medicine's gaze from locating disease in individual bodies, and all the individuating effects that follow from this, to locating the pathological across different bodies and *in* the family.

They also do more than this. In the place of contemporary forms of medical disposal and decision-making, in which the display of expertise entails speedy closure, what is found in the genetic clinic is a slowing down of clinic process, and explicit moments of undecidability, uncertainty and instability over genetic diagnostic categories. Equally, and at the same time, a firm commitment to the possibility of certainty, of fixing diagnostic categories in grids and codes through the future development of technoscience, is also implicitly being performed.

Thus dysmorphology helps us to see how the clinic is a centre of not only calculation but also discretion. Even where there are tests, dysmorphology performs clinical judgement as deciding whether or not a test result is accurate or salient. Furthermore, by maintaining uncertainty dysmorphology also legitimates the need for more genetic-technoscience, and more clinical judgement in the future to help fix diagnostic possibilities.

Medicine's humanism

> The constant division between the normal and the abnormal, to which every individual is subjected, brings us back to our own time, by applying the binary branding and exile of the leper to quite different objects; the existence of a whole set of techniques and institutions for measuring, supervising and correcting the abnormal brings into play the disciplinary mechanisms to which the fear of the plague gave rise. All the mechanisms of power, which, even today, are disposed around the abnormal individual, to brand him and to alter him, are composed of those two forms from which they distantly derive.
>
> (Foucault 1995)

A medical way has very specific features. Firstly, it is a way of conceiving the body as *an object to be known:* this legitimates examination and entry *into* the body to make it visible. Young (1997) helps us to see how this process, and the complicity of the patient in it, is still performed by the clinic:

> the history-taking is still the realm of the self, though one in which the self is becoming detached from the body, the physical examination is a realm of the body, and one in which the body is rendered an object.
>
> (p.26)

Secondly, the body is conceived of as both organic and machine-like, made up of functional parts, whose malfunctioning legitimates intervention in the body.

The body is often imagined within the bio-physiological mechanical model as a functional machine needing fixes to its parts and its ills. That the detection and the cure of disease is possible (provided the right way to knowledge is followed) legitimates particular interventions, particular forms of experimentation, and of course the need for more technology to help make the body and its ever smaller parts visible to the gaze.

But the anatomy and the physiology of the body in medicine are also dividing practices that define *the normal* and identify *deviations* from the normal. These are not value neutral: 'medicine formulates the human body and disease in a *culturally distinctive fashion*' (Good 1997, p.65, emphasis added) and in ways which are *normative.*

Here there is real slippage in the notion of normativity. Canguilhem (1991) suggests that in medicine the '[n]ormative in the fullest sense of the word, is that which establishes norms' (p.127). It is a vital principle of living organisms to maintain life (see also Greco 2009). But what many theorists have shown, after Foucault, is how in medicine there is slippage between this sense of normativity and a moral or ethical sense of normativity, through which the normal becomes both a quality of the person and a reference point or 'standard', or critically does not. Capturing some of this in his discussion of the anthropological problem of the relation between the social body and the biological body in medicine, Taussig (1980) argues that medical knowledge is not just culturally constructed. Rather, medical knowledge as it describes and treats is constitutive of cultural values and social relations.

What gets hidden, Taussig is suggesting, are not only the social relations that create a disease, such as poverty and exploitation. The very language of disease – that which constitutes diseases as if they are naturally occurring phenomena – conceals the social relations that have gone into the making of this language, into the making of the specific diseases. This includes ways in which some attributes are valued over others to create the very standards and norms upon which the creation of the pathological, of diseases, depends.

These standards and norms once reified appear as objective facts, not as creations that embed value. For example, cultural notions of what does or does not count as brainpower informs the standards by which what does and does not count as a healthy brain are measured. Where a person deviates from these standards they are also vulnerable to being devalued, because they are being rendered as deviating from, or even transgressing, cultural conceptions of what it is to be a full person, or even human. Within this perspective medicine is a site of biopolitics in which difference can be recast as abnormality, as unnatural and even as pathological.

Dysmorphology and deferral

With hindsight dysmorphology has proved to be an obvious site in which to study the relation between the new genetics and medicine. Yet what the study has uncovered is that this relation is far from straightforward. To the contrary, dysmorphology performs an unanticipated need for clinical discretion in the production of genetic knowledge. Specifically, dysmorphology draws together conventional clinical methods and techniques with new ways of thinking about the origins of abnormality and pathology to reinvigorate the substantive importance of the clinical gaze. In the various ways delineated in the study, dysmorphology performs the clinic as critical to the production not just the consumption of medical knowledge. As an emergent category and system of classification, the genetic is performed in dysmorphology as *needing* clinical judgement in the work of distinguishing the genetic from the non-genetic.

Genetic science thus emerges as a new frontier, in which so much is not yet known or not yet standardized. Here I suggest, tentatively and provisionally, how undecidability, uncertainty and instability of genetic diagnosis – as prominent features of clinical practice in dysmorphology – perform something about the genetic clinic that is highly significant. This sustained pressure of ambiguity and uncertainty requires additional explanation when it runs alongside a firm commitment to a future of diagnostic certainty. In this view it is precisely those moments of ambiguity and uncertainty that help to *make a space of deferral*. The clinic holds patients and parents on the genetic ground and establishes the very space of deferral which is needed to secure that future: a future in which classification becomes sedimented in a technoscience that will continue to press back the boundaries of the genomic unknown, but a technoscience that also creates opportunities for more clinical judgement to secure its proper interpretation and salience. Here I need to elaborate.

The point is to suggest how members in the clinic create a space of deferral in which the genetic itself is performed as very much still open, and its categories as revisable. Thus the dysmorphology clinic emerges as a site in which we can observe the complex, practical work of classification. Clinical uncertainty and the trope of deferral mean that the logic of the clinic appears to call for advances in technoscience that foreshadow its own demise. This is the way of the clinic. Clinical findings are legitimated by the outcomes of laboratory genetic science. The clinic performs an apparent commitment to future facts that are secured in the laboratory. But this projection is itself always being deferred. This deferral creates the space in which the clinic and pathological entities are irreducible to mere data, to codes and numbers, including molecular biology. Thus the colonization and subjection of the clinic augured by commentators such as Rose (2006) is premature. Rather, the clinic in dysmorphology is being reperformed as a site of knowledge production in the identification and classification of genetic pathologies.

Alignments and power

The question that arises then is not that of settling the matter of medical dominance as if this was an abstract issue pure and simple. The issue is more one of understanding how and when medicine exercises its authority and discretion.

The territory I have explored in the book is how and when does medicine maintain its dominance even in the context of apparent challenges to its professional powers, the proliferation of technosciences such as the new genetics, and the deconstruction of a standard, normal and natural body that undermines its statistical base in fact rather than fiction. How is it that medicine keeps going even in the face of all its apparent technological, epistemological and ontological failure? And, crucially, what is the place of the clinic in all this?

Central to this more subtle and intricate thesis of medical dominance is a reconsideration of the relationship between power, medicine and society. While acknowledging earlier accounts of biomedical dominance, the perspective I offer depends upon investigating the clinic as a 'complex location' (Cooper 1997 in Latimer 2000). Specifically, the clinic in this perspective is treated both as a discursive space that has system properties and as a site of culture through which it works as a social institution.

My particular focus is not to offer a political economy of the medical profession's dominance, or chart its decline, after Navarro (1988) or Willis (2006), although I hope what I have shown goes some way to helping us understand how it is possible for medicine to be so deeply implicated across very different and disparate political economies enlisted as a senior partner of post-genomic 'biocapitalism' (Kaushik 2006). Instead, I have updated emphases in earlier accounts of medicine as a social institution by drawing together a theoretical framework that offers a more contemporary understanding of power.

Specifically, I have shown how medicine keeps its dominant place alive through its alignments, extensions, disposals, attachments and detachments, as well as extends its power through the specificities of its associations with the new genetics, including new forms of biopower that individuate society into persons. But alongside this I have also underlined those moments that undermine the dominant figure of the individual, if temporarily, so that it is medicine that has to rescue persons from the inchoate of being merely DNA and return them to forms of being human that make people much more than the sum of their bodily parts, including their genotype.

In this medicine is not so much dominating through the heroics of intervention and cure, and the accomplishment of 'medical miracles' (Becker 1993). Rather what we have seen is a shift from heroic, functional medicine, healing the sick and 'raising the dead' (Becker 1993), back to the clinic as the site of scientific medicine involved in classification, discretion and the biopolitics of selection. Nonetheless medicine remains a site where classification, and participation in the clinical work of categorizing people's troubles, acts as a form of intervention. What we have seen is an extension of medicine's power in which representing is a form of intervention, one that has the potential to not simply put right something that is wrong with a person's body or mind, but one that gets at the very fabric of what people are made of to change how they think of themselves and their children and their family at the most basic of levels.

I am suggesting therefore a very different way of looking at medicine. As discussed above, earlier theorists explored how management technologies can each be considered in terms of posing challenges to medical authority and power. These technologies have included financial and management accounting, the rise of patient consumerism and the widening of access to medical information and knowledge, the proliferation of technoscientific knowledge and alternative conceptualizations of the body as well as the meanings of health and illness. Instead of seeing these as competing technologies, I am arguing that the very processes and practices that seem to challenge medicine, such as genetic science and technology, can on closer inspection be seen to become, intermittently, medicine's extensions and allies, and do so in ways that magnify and enhance, rather than undermine clinical authority, particularly at the opening up of a new frontier.

In the past, I have analysed how attempts to make medicine more accountable through introduction of management technologies do not so much challenge medical power, but provide available grounds with which medicine can intermittently align in unexpected ways to reproduce its dominant position (Latimer 1999, 2000, 2004). In the current analysis it is the very intermittency and partiality of the interaction of the gene and the clinic, as well as the incompleteness of the phenotype–genotype relation that helps mobilize, translate and revive medicine's place.

Working society

There is little doubt that medicine's history is one of association and alignment, rather than, as Freidson (1988) suggested, of closure and purity. Yet the present study indicates its dominance today arises as much from its readiness to work *partial* associations and *momentary* alignments, and to do so intermittently.

The fourth part of the book, 'The Family and Identities', continues this theme by elaborating how family are enrolled in the clinic in ways that help institute the clinic as both a site of science in the description and classification of genetic aberrations, and as a centre of calculation in the management of the reproduction of abnormal forms. Here I have shown how the clinic in dysmorphology attaches intermittently to the family and plays into and out of discourses of parenting and nurture as a site accountable for the healthy bodies and development of children. So while I have also suggested the clinic is concerned with disorders of the body that imply long-term, sometimes disabling conditions, it does more than this.

Chapters 9, 10 and 11, as I detail further below, show how the clinic's access to and enrolment of the family allows the clinic to become a different kind of laboratory, one in which the relationship between genetic aberrations, the social relations of reproduction and aberrations in human development and form are being observed and classified. Here the clinic because of its immersion in families can do what laboratory-based science cannot. It can trace, describe and classify the effects that are the consequence of who marries and procreates with who. Thus the clinic in dysmorphology is the site of a 'naturalist science', in which humans, rather than plants or animals, as they engage in sexual reproduction are the subjects observed and classified into syndromes.

In accomplishing this work, the clinic begins by assessing the risk of the presenting condition, in terms of prognosis, as well as in terms of recurrence in future pregnancies and other family members. It makes family aware of itself as just that, family, and of how not only lifestyle needs to be managed in the production of healthy citizens for the future, but nature itself requires management, because nature is risky. Indeed it is society's need for genetic counselling to manage the reproduction of children with long-term and often disabling conditions that gives the clinic as a site of science access to families, and vice versa. Family are enrolled through careful and long-winded processes of attachment, including helping to recover the humanity of the genetically aberrant as well as parents' face.

In Chapter 9 I explored the effects of clinical practices in terms of the kinds of persons being produced and reproduced by clinical processes and practices. I discussed contemporary debate over postmodern biology that augurs the destruction of the humanist individual. However rather than the totalizing effects of a geneticization of the body that destroys the figure of children as individuals, I showed how through a shift in ground, children are rehumanized as much more than the effect of a syndrome. Through refiguring them as people who need to know and who are capable of knowledge as well as agentic and wilful, their Euro-American personhood is, for a moment, reinstated. As such medicine reinstitutes syndromes and bodies as the effects of a genotype–phenotype relation, while they as persons are refigured as the complex figures of humanist thought whose consciousness, or mind, is able to detach from and be elevated over their body. Medicine thus reasserts its own humanity in ways that help attach it to the family. Specifically, paediatric genetic medicine, in all its crossings, reperforms the clinic as at the 'pinnacle' of the human rather than the life sciences.

Chapter 10 revisited the relationship between medicine and the family, particularly in the context of contemporary discourses that institute parenting as an extension of actor-networks of public health. Specifically, moments of prediction and calculation are arrived at during processes of diagnosis. In dysmorphology, these moments are 'occasioned' by these diagnostic processes; they are not managed by clinical staff as discrete events. And parents and other family members are encouraged, from the home visit through to clinical consultations, to participate in these knowledge practices. Hence, the alignment of the gene and the clinic in dysmorphology creates access to the family as a site of reproduction of these long-term, chronic conditions and allows medicine to intervene in this site.

In all this I showed how the bodies of children become the visible manifestation and measure of good parenting, in terms of looking good, being good and being healthy. However I also discussed how good parenting in these discourses is directed at lifestyle choice. I then went on to explore what family becomes in the genetics clinic and how at the same time as clinical processes intensify the responsibalization of parents as reproducing the future of healthy progeny, the alignment of the genetic clinic and the family institutes parents not merely as agents providing the right kind of environment for their child, but as family members whose biological matter may or may not need reforming. I thus argued that the family gets reinstalled in genetic medicine as a site of selection. Within this perspective individuals are not constituted as 'prepatients' (Konrad 2005) but as 'future parents', whose future acts of procreation may or may not produce genetically aberrant children. Genetic counselling emerges in these discourses as processes of interaction with the family through which the biological substance of the family, and thus the shape and form of its individual members, can be reformed.

In Chapter 11, I focussed on these interactions in the clinic and on parents' accounts of their experiences of encounters with genetic medicine. Examining consultations between families and clinicians, I showed that family members are not so much disciplined in these encounters but are enrolled in the everyday work of clinical differentiation. Thus the mechanisms through which the abnormal is classified and disciplined are extended in genetic medicine from the individual to the family. It is only by extending its existing alignment with the family that clinical medicine makes itself an 'obligatory passage' (Latour 1987) to the new genetics. Specifically, dysmorphology not only helps to create a new space of medical intervention in the management of long-term, chronic conditions through mediating their reproduction, it installs itself through deferral and undecideability as at the heart of the classification of the relation between the genetic and the pathological.

In this context I interrogated the nature and extent of family participation to show how interactions between the clinic and the family constitute relations of exchange, in which family members gift the clinic access to the family, both virtual and literal, in the form of bodies, photographs, histories and accounts. In exchange parents are given a perspective, a way to knowledge that gives hope of a future of classification for what is wrong with their child/family. Specifically, family members are not simply informed about 'what is', rather, the clinic becomes a site of gathering, which engages parents in the epistemological work of objectification and differentiation, through which what is unusual or abnormal about their child and other family members, including themselves, is defined alongside clinician's performance of deferral. The chapter showed how participation in this motility of clinical work moves parents between definition and deferral to excite consciousness of the riskiness of reproduction, elicit moments of reflexivity and accomplish shifts in perspective.

The clinic in dysmorphology is thus performed as a space in which medicine, aligned with genetics, can help to make a difference to the future shape of a family, and therefore of society. Medical intervention here does not, as we have seen, involve direct action on the genes. This is not a site of genetic engineering, although the work of dysmorphology does help to legitimate the need for technology with which to engineer the genetically aberrant in the future. Rather it creates a space that problematizes reproduction as a possible source of particular kinds of chronic conditions. Reproduction here doubles for cellular reproduction and sexual reproduction. Intervention consists of modes of representation or 'genetic counselling' that mediates how people imagine the effects of their procreative relations and excites consciousness of the need for them to manage their reproductive lives reflexively.

Whatever else can be said about it, dysmorphology in the end is about the study of the misshapen. So it gets to the heart of much of the preoccupation over identity and belonging that drives contemporary consumption. Its field of operation, as I have been indicating throughout is the work of distinguishing the normal from the abnormal body, at both the level of the body's surfaces as well as of its invisible spaces. Dysmorphology is thus a site that helps to institute a new relation between abnormality and its causes.

In the contemporary clinic, rather than notions of sin, it is parental lifestyle and neonatal environment as well genes that provide the grounds of explanation for dysmorphias. Each of these possible grounds shifts the relation between biology, nature, human agency and reproduction. Neither God, the soul nor the supernatural play much of a part in the dysmorphology clinic. Rather the very etymology of the word dysmorphology as well as its practices help to put into play a different set of relations: these help reproduce what constitutes the abnormal as well as circulate new ways of thinking about the causes of abnormality and deformity.

Critically, dysmorphology then is a site in which we can see how the work of geneticizing certain conditions sanitises the marking of the abnormal, making it ethically acceptable. In a cultural context which celebrates diversity and difference and in which the very notion of a normal body is being problematized this is an especially important part of the work that genetic medicine does because it helps legitimate both the consumption and the disposal of the genetically aberrant. Thus genetic medicine in dysmorphology is different from that critiqued by Taussig and others cited in the Introduction. Specifically, dysmorphology *needs* to make explicit the social relations of reproduction as creating congenital abnormalities. And sensitivity to difference is a fundamental aspect of the dysmorphology gaze, one that helps both divide off and also reinclude the most genetically aberrant in the fold of the human.

Through switches in ground and attachment to the family and the fleshy bodies of babies, children and their families, dysmorphology gives presence to them as human, as much more than the sum of their bodily parts. We have seen how this affirmation holds children so easily reconstituted as killable in the fold of the human, and reinstates medicine as itself on the side of humanity, thus reaffirming its own humanism in terms of the detachment of consciousness. This said we have also seen how at other moments, as in the case of Johnny, clinicians do not hesitate to consider putting a stop on the reproduction of children such as Johnny. But as I have discussed the kind of human beings being distinguished and affirmed by the clinic is itself exclusive: it is a human being celebrated by enlightenment humanism, and as such it cuts out other perspectives on what it is to be human.

Notes

1 Introduction

1 All names given in interviews and extracts from field notes throughout the book are fictitious.

3 Medicalizing science

1 There is a wonderful wood engraving of an alchemist's laboratory in Petrach's *Phisicke Against Fortune* by Weiditz, Hans, the Younger (um 1500–1536), created in 1532 (http://www.fine-art-images.net/en/showIMG_11647.html Accessed February 2012).

4 The 'translation' of growth and form

1 In using the term deep play I am drawing on Clifford Geertz's essay (1973) on the Balinese cockfight, who in turn borrows the notion from Jeremy Bentham (1748–1832), a British philosopher and social reformer. This genealogy of the term is particularly apposite as Bentham was the spiritual founder of University College, London, the home university of Professor Smart and the London Dysmorphology Club, and whose medical school was also home to Bentham's model for the panoptic prison when I trained there in 1977.
2 This original work formed the basis of a classificatory system that is continuously added to and updated – OMIM (Online Mendelian Inheritance in Man)® http://www.ncbi.nlm. nih.gov/omim
3 I have not the space to explore these kinds of technologies fully. This has been done elsewhere, for example Newman (1996).
4 'Karyotype: A photomicrograph of an individual's *chromosomes* arranged in a standard format showing the number, size, and shape of each chromosome type; used in low-resolution *physical mapping* to correlate gross chromosomal abnormalities with the characteristics of specific diseases.' http://www.ornl.gov/sci/techresources/Human_ Genome/glossary/glossary_k.shtml

5 Shaping the science of growth and form

1 'The name "Charge" was a clever way (in 1981) to refer to a newly recognized cluster of features seen in a number of children. Over the years, it has become clear that Charge is indeed a syndrome and at least one gene causing Charge syndrome has been discovered (see below). The letters in Charge stand for: Coloboma of the eye, Heart defects, Atresia of the choanae, Retardation of growth and/or development, Genital and/or urinary

abnormalities, and **E**ar abnormalities and deafness. Those features are no longer used in making a diagnosis of Charge syndrome, but we're not changing the name.' (http://chargesyndrome.org/about-charge.asp Accessed September 2011)

2 Hans Gruneberg, 'distinguished for his work on animal genetics in relation to medicine', died in 1983. He worked at Medical Research Council Group for Experimental Research in Inherited Diseases, University College London (BMJ 1983, p.137).

3 http://oxgrid.angis.org.au/mouse/human/500_index.html (Accessed May 2010).

4 A knock-out mouse is a transgenic mouse with a deleted gene – it is an engineered mutant, unlike the Bleb mutant mice, which are 'naturally' occuring.

6 Creating clinical pictures

1 Photographs are one of the immutable mobiles (Latour 1987, p.227) through which the signs (or *absence* of signs) of dysmorphia are inscribed and circulated. The significance of how diagnostic work in dysmorphology constitutes and disposes of slides and photographs is discussed at greater length elsewhere (see Featherstone *et al.* 2005; Latimer *et al.* 2006; Shaw *et al.* 2003).

7 Rebirthing the clinic

1 'Velo-Cardio-Facial Syndrome is an autosomal dominant condition. Genetic studies of children with this condition show that a microscopic segment on the long arm of chromosome 22 is missing. The genetic test for diagnosis of this condition is called "FISH analysis" and can be performed in many medical centers.' (http://www.faces-cranio.org/Disord/Velo.htm Accessed June 2011)

2 'Marfan syndrome is a genetic (inherited) condition that affects the body's connective tissues. Connective tissues provide support and structure to other tissue and organs. The symptoms of Marfan syndrome vary from person to person, as the condition can affect the connective tissues in different areas of the body. For example, it can affect: blood vessels, causing damage to the heart; skeleton, causing long, thin limbs; eyes, causing the lens (the transparent structure at the front of the eye) to fall into an abnormal position (lens dislocation)' http://www.nhs.uk/conditions/Marfan-syndrome/Pages/Introduction.aspx (Accessed June 2012).

3 During this period research was being undertaken that challenged the clinical picture of Marfan syndrome in ways that was revising its 'nosology' to put more emphasis on heart problems and the confirmatory FISH test than on the overgrowth of bone (Loeys *et al.* 2010).

8 Dysmorphology's portraits

1 T. Sydenham, quoted by F. Boissier de Sauvages (1772) *Nosologie methodique*, vol. 1, Lyons. p.88.

2 I am grateful to Paul Atkinson for some of this detail over the history of photographs in medical work. See also Featherstone *et al.* (2005).

3 Just to remind the reader, chromosomes carry up to 4,220 genes apiece.

9 Genes, bodies, persons

1 Propagules in sexual reproduction are seeds.

2 As Lange (2003) in her essay on Aristotle's biology notes, in the phallocentric worldview there is a conflation of male and human, with woman's biology rendering her animal and irrational.

3 Agamben (2002) draws attention to a double paradox here – classical and medieval religious texts portray how at the moment of their return to paradise humans are restored as animal, because it is their consciousness that is both a cause and effect of their fall from grace.
4 The clinic has long been a site in which body–self relations have been performed. As Leder (1990) asserts, in many ways the body in medicine as lived is absent, except as a corpse. Rather, the body is only interesting clinically as site for the location of disease.
5 In a conversation with Paul Rabinow I began to understand how Haraway's project in *When Species Meet* (2007) could be understood as a manifesto of connectivity with non-humans that brings them into the fold of the best of humanist thought and institutions.

11 Transforming family

1 Thanks to Marilyn Strathern for this observation.
2 There is some evidence in the study that suggests that to be fully included in the clinic parents need to demonstrate their *commitment* to finding out about their child's condition, indeed this seems, from informal conversations with practitioners, to be one of the things that the specialist nurses as well as the doctors are, as Dr Smith puts it, 'sussing out' (see also White *et al.* 2012).
3 'Neuronal migration disorder which results in broad, flattened gyri and occasionally is described as incomplete lissencephaly. Typically, children have developmental delay and seizures, the onset and severity depending on the severity of the cortical malformation. Infantile spasms are common in affected children, as is intractable epilepsy. In some patients there are mutations of chromosome 17 and Xq22 but others will have no specific chromosomal marker. Those with chromosome 17 mutations more frequently have areas of pachygyria in the frontal and temporal regions, whereas those with Xq22 abnormalities often have abnormalities in the frontal lobe.' http://www. amershamhealth.com/medcyclopaedia/medical/Volume%20VII/PACHYGYRIA.asp (Accessed October 2011).
4 'Noonan syndrome was first recognized as a unique entity in 1963 when Noonan and Ehmke described a series of patients with unusual faces and multiple malformations, including congenital heart disease. These patients were previously thought to have a form of Turner syndrome, with which Noonan syndrome shares a number of clinical features. The observation that patients with Noonan syndrome have normal karyotypes was important in allowing the distinction to be made between the Turner and Noonan syndromes. The cardinal features of Noonan syndrome are unusual faces (ie, hypertelorism, down-slanting eyes, webbed neck), congenital heart disease (in 50%), short stature, and chest deformity. Approximately 25% of individuals with Noonan syndrome have mental retardation. Bleeding diathesis is present in as many as half of all patients with Noonan syndrome. Skeletal, neurologic, genitourinary, lymphatic, eye, and skin findings may be present to varying degrees. **Pathophysiology:** The pathophysiology of Noonan syndrome is not fully understood. Linkage analysis performed on a Dutch family with autosomal dominant Noonan syndrome suggested that a gene for Noonan syndrome is on chromosome arm 12q. **Frequency: In the US:** The incidence of Noonan syndrome is estimated at 1 in 1000 to 1 in 2500 live births. **Internationally:** The incidence of Noonan syndrome appears to be consistent worldwide. **Mortality/ Morbidity:** The primary source of morbidity and mortality in these patients depends on the presence and type of congenital heart disease. **Race:** Noonan syndrome is panethnic. **Sex:** Noonan syndrome occurs in either a sporadic or autosomal dominant fashion. In either case, males and females are affected equally. **Age:** The disorder is present from birth, but age impacts upon the facial phenotype. Infants with Noonan syndrome can be difficult to recognize by facial appearance alone. The phenotype becomes more striking in early childhood, but with advancing age, it may again become quite subtle. Careful

examination of an affected child's parents may in fact reveal that they are affected mildly.' http://www.emedicine.com/PED/topic1616.htm (Accessed September 2005).

5 Human Doublecortin, an x-linked gene located on Xq chromosome, first reported in 1998. Mutations of this gene have been linked with lissencephaly, a brain disorder that results in epilepsy and developmental delay.

6 'Branchiootorenal (BOR) syndrome is an autosomal dominant condition characterized by ear abnormalities, hearing loss, cysts in the neck, and kidney problems. Description: The name "branchiootorenal syndrome" describes the body systems most commonly affected by this genetic disorder. The term "branchio" refers to the abnormalities of the neck found in individuals with this syndrome. Cysts (lump or swelling that can be filled with fluid) and fistulas (abnormal passage from the throat to the skin) in the neck occur frequently. The term "oto" refers to the ear disorders associated with the syndrome. For example, the outer ear can be unusual in appearance. Hearing loss is also common. Finally, the term "renal" stands for the kidney problems commonly seen in patients with this condition. These can be very mild or very severe, as can any of the symptoms associated with this disorder. Dr. M. Melnick first described branchiootorenal syndrome in 1975. Another name for BOR syndrome is Melnick-Fraser syndrome. Individuals with BOR syndrome typically have physical differences that are present at birth (congenital). These birth defects are caused by a change (mutation) in a gene.' http://health.enotes.com/genetic-disorders-encyclopedia/branchiootorenal-syndrome#Definition (Accessed December 2005).

Bibliography

Aase, J.M. (1990) *Diagnostic Dysmorphology*. New York: Plenum Medical.

Agamben, G. (2002) *The Open: Man and Animal*. Translated by Giorgio Agamben and Kevin Attell. Stanford: Stanford University Press.

Alcoff, L. (undated) Foucault's Philosophy of Science: Structures of Truth/Structures of Power. http://www.alcoff.com/content/foucphi.html (Accessed January 2011).

Altman, L.K. (2006) Socratic Dialogue Gives Way to PowerPoint. *New York Times*. 12 December, p.F1.

The American College of Medical Genetics (2006) Newborn Screening: Toward a Uniform Screening Panel and System. *Genetics in Medicine*, 8 (5): 1–14.

Appleyard, B. (2012) Not in Our Genes. *Sunday Times*, 17 June.

Arksey, H. (1994) Expert and Lay Participation in the Construction of Medical Knowledge. *Sociology of Health and Illness*, 16: 448–68.

Armstrong, D. (1983a) *Political Anatomy of the Body: Medical Knowledge in Britain in the Twentieth Century*. Cambridge: Cambridge University Press.

Armstrong, D. (1983b) The New Hygiene of the Dispensary. In D. Armstrong (Ed.) *Political Anatomy of the Body: Medical Knowledge in Britain in the Twentieth Century*. Cambridge: Cambridge University Press. pp.7–18.

Armstrong, D. (1995) The Rise of Surveillance Medicine. *Sociology of Health & Illness*, 17 (3): 393–404.

Armstrong, D. (2002) Clinical Autonomy, Individual and Collective: The Problem of Changing Doctors' Behaviour. *Social Science and Medicine*, 55 (10): 1771–7.

Armstrong, D. (2007) Professionalism, Indeterminacy and the EBM Project. *BioSocieties*, 2: 73–84.

Atkinson, P. (1995) *Medical Talk and Medical Work*. London: Sage.

Atkinson, P. (1997) *The Clinical Experience: The Construction and Reconstruction of Medical Reality*. 2nd edition. Aldershot, Hants: Ashgate.

Atkinson P., Glasner, P. and Greenslade, H. (2006) *New Genetics, New Identities*. London: Routledge.

Atkinson, P., Parsons, E. and Featherstone, K. (2001) Professional Constructions of Family and Kinship in Medical Genetics. *New Genetics and Society*, 20 (1): 5–24.

Atkinson, P., Reid, M. and Sheldrake, P. (1977) Medical Mystique Part 1: Indeterminacy and Professional Process; Part 2: Case studies in professional process. *Sociology of Work and Occupations*, 4 (3): 243–80.

Attard, M. (2009) *Carriers of Responsibility*. PhD thesis. University of Sydney.

Ballard, K. and Elston, M.A. (2005) Medicalization: A Multi-Dimensional Concept. *Social Theory and Health*, 3 (3): 228–41.

Barnes, B. (1988) *The Nature of Power*. Cambridge: Polity Press.

Barnes, B. (2005) Elusive Memories of Technoscience. *Perspectives on Science*, 13 (2): 142–65.

Bauman, Z. (1989) *Modernity and the Holocaust*. Cambridge: Polity Press.

Bauman, Z. (1990) Effacing the Face: on the Social Management of Moral Proximity. *Theory, Culture and Society*, 7 (1): 5–38.

Bauman, Z. (1991) The Social Manipulation of Morality: Moralizing Actors, Adiaphorising Action. *Theory, Culture and Society*, 8 (1): 137–51.

Bauman, Z. (1995) *Life in Fragments: Essays in Post-Modern Morality*. Oxford: Blackwell.

Bauman, Z. (2003) *Liquid Love: On the Frailty of Human Bonds*. Cambridge: Polity Press.

BBSRC (Biotechnology and Biological Sciences Research Council) (undated) Our Vision. http://www.bbsrc.ac.uk/organisation/vision.aspx (Accessed February 2012).

Beck-Gershwein, E. (2002) *Reinventing the Family: In Search of New Lifestyles*. Translated by Patrick Camiller. Cambridge: Polity Press.

Becker, H.S. (1993) How I Learned What a Crock Was. *Journal of Contemporary Ethnography*, 22: 28–35.

Bellam, M. and Vijeratnam, S. (2012) From child health surveillance to child health promotion, and onwards: a tale of babies and bathwater. *Archives of Disease in Childhood*, 97: 73–7.

Berg, M. (1992) The Construction of Medical Disposals. Medical Sociology and Medical Problem-Solving in Clinical Practice. *Sociology of Health and Illness*, 14 (2): 151–80.

Berg, M. (1997) *Rationalising Medical Work*. Cambridge MA: MIT Press.

Bharadwaj, A. (2002) Uncertain Risk: Genetic Screening for Susceptibility to Haemochromatosis. *Health, Risk and Society*, 4 (3): 227–40.

Biehl, J. and Moran-Thomas, A. (2009) Symptom: Subjectivities, Social Ills, Technologies. *Annual Review of Anthropology*, 38: 267–88.

Birenbaum, A. (1992) Courtesy stigma revisited. *Mental Retardation*, 30 (5): 265–8.

Birke, L. (1998) The Broken Heart. In M. Shildrick and J. Price (Eds) *Vital signs: Feminist Reconfigurations of the Bio/logical Body*. Edinburgh: Edinburgh University Press. pp.197–223.

Black, D. (2011) What Is a Face? *Body & Society*, December, 17: 1–25.

Bloor, M. and McIntosh, J. (1990) Surveillance and concealment: a comparison of client resistance in therapeutic communities and health visiting. In S. Cunningham- Burley and N.P. McKeganey (Eds) *Readings in Medical Sociology*. London: Routledge. pp.159–81.

B.M.J. (British Medical Journal) (1983) Professor Hans Grüneberg. Obituary. *British Medical Journal*, 286: 137.

Bouquet, M. (1994) Family Trees and their Affinities: The Visual Imperative of the Genealogical Diagram. *Journal of the Royal Anthropological Institute, (N.S.)*, 2 (1): 43–66.

Bourdieu, P. (1977) *Outline of a Theory of Practice*. Cambridge: Cambridge University Press.

Bourdieu, P. (1984) *Distinction. A Social Critique of the Judgement of Taste*. Translated by Richard Nice. Boston, MA: Harvard University Press.

Bowker, G. and Star, L. (2000) *Sorting Things Out*. Cambridge, MA: MIT Press.

Bramwell, R., West, H. and Salmon, P. (2006) Health Professionals' and Service Users' Interpretation of Screening Test Results: Experimental Study. *British Medical Journal*, 333 (7566): 468.

Brighton, P. and Brighton, G. (1987) *The Man Behind the Syndrome*. New York: Springer.

Brodwin, P. (2002) Genetics, Identity and the Anthropology of Essentialism. *Anthropology Quarterly*, 75 (2): 323–30.

Broussard, L. (2011) From the Lab to the Clinic and Back: Translational Research Training and Careers. *Science Careers*, http://sciencecareers.sciencemag.org/career_magazine/previous_issues/articles/2011_05_13/science.opms.r1100103 (Accessed December 2011).

Brown, N. and Webster, A. (2004) *New Medical Technologies and Society: Reordering Life*. Cambridge: Polity Press.

Brush, P. (1998) Metaphors of Inscription: Discipline, Plasticity and the Rhetoric of Choice. *Feminist Review*, 58: 22–43.

Bury, M. and Taylor, D. (2008) Towards a Theory of Care Transition: From Medical Dominance to Managed Consumerism. *Social Theory and Health*, 6 (3): 201–19.

Callon, M. (1986) Some elements of a sociology of translation: domestication of the scallops and the fishermen of St Brieuc Bay. In J. Law (Ed.) *Power, action and belief: a new sociology of knowledge?* London: Routledge. pp.196–223.

Callon, M. (2006) Papier Recherche de CSI. No: 005. What Does it Mean to Say that Economics is Performative? http://halshs.archives-ouvertes.fr/docs/00/09/15/96/PDF/WP_CSI_005.pdf (Accessed January 2012).

Callon, M. and Rabeharisoa, V. (2003) Research 'in the wild' and the shaping of new social identities. *Technology in Society*, 25: 193–204.

Callon, M. and Rabeharisoa, V. (2008) The Growing Engagement of Emergent Concerned Groups in Political and Economic Life: Lessons from the French Association of Neuromuscular Disease Patients. *Science, Technology & Human Values*, 33 (2): 230–61.

Cambrosio, A., Guttman, R.D. and Keating, P. (1994) New Medical Technologies and Clinical Practice: A Survey of Lymphocyte Subset Monitoring. *Clinical Transplantation*, 8: 532–40.

Canguilhem, G. (1991) *The Normal and the Pathological*. Translated by C.R. Fawcett and R.S. Cohen. New York: Zone Books.

Carroll, S.B. (2005) *Endless Forms Most Beautiful*. New York: Norton & Co.

Carsten, J. (Ed.) (2000) *Cultures of Relatedness: New Approaches to the Study of Kinship*. Cambridge: Cambridge University Press.

Carsten, J. (2004) *After Kinship*. Cambridge: Cambridge University Press.

Chadwick, R. (1992) Having Children. In R. Chadwick (Ed.) *Ethics, Reproduction and Genetic Control*. London: Routledge. pp.3–48.

Charon, R. and Wyer, P. (2008) Narrative Evidence Based Medicine, for the NEBM Working Group. *The Lancet*, 371 (9609): 296–7.

Chatterji, R., Chattoo, S. and Das, V.A. (1998) The Death of the Clinic? Normality and Pathology in Recrafting Aging Bodies. In M. Shildrick and J. Price (Eds) *Vital signs: Feminist Reconfigurations of the Bio/logical Body*. Edinburgh: Edinburgh University Press. pp.171–96.

Clarke, A. (1991) Non-Directive Genetic Counselling. *The Lancet*, 338 (8781): 1524.

Clarke, A.E. (1998) *Disciplining Reproduction: Modernity, American Life Sciences and the 'Problems of Sex'*. Berkeley: University of California Press.

Clarke, A.E. (2005) *Situational Analysis: Grounded Theory After The Postmodern Turn*. Thousand Oaks, CA: Sage.

Clarke, A.E., Shim J.K., Mamo, L., Fosket, J.R. and Fishman J.R. (2003) Biomedicalization: Technoscientific transformations of health, illness, and U.S. biomedicine. *American Sociological Review*, 68 (2): 161–94.

Clarke, A.E., Shim, J., Mamo, L., Fosket, J. and Fishman, J. (Eds) (2010) *Biomedicalization: Technoscience and Transformations of Health and Illness in the United States*. Durham, NC: Duke University Press.

Clarke, J. (undated) Does the shape of my face show that I have a genetic disorder? *How Stuff Works*. http://science.howstuffworks.com/environmental/life/genetic/dysmorphology1. htm (Accessed November 2011).

Clegg, S.R. (1989) *Frameworks of Power*. London: Sage.

Coffin-Lowry Syndrome Foundation (undated) Welcome to the Coffin-Lowry Syndrome Foundation. http://clsf.info/ (Accessed November 2011).

Cohen, A.P. (1992) Post-Fieldwork Fieldwork. *Journal of Anthropological Research*, 48 (4): 339–54.

Cohen, J. and Meskin, A. (2004) On the Epistemic Value of Photographs. *The Journal of Aesthetics and Art Criticism*. Special Issue: Art, Mind, and Cognitive Science, 62 (2): 197–210.

Coleman, B. (2006) What is genomics and post genomics? Natural Environment Research Council. http://www.nerc.ac.uk/research/programmes/proteomics/background/whatis. asp (Accessed February 2012).

Collier, S.J. and Ong, A. (2005) Global Assemblages, Anthropological Problems. In A. Ong and S.J. Collier (Eds), *Global Assemblages: Technology, Politics, and Ethics as Anthropological Problems*. Malden, MA: Blackwell. pp.3–22.

Condit, C.M. (1999) The Meanings of the Gene. *Public Debates about Human Heredity*. Madison, Wisconsin: University of Wisconsin Press.

Conrad, P. (1999) A mirage of genes. *Sociology of Health & Illness*, 21 (2): 228–41.

Cooke-Deegan, R. (2003) Past Promises and Future Realities. Keynote Paper, Trading Genes: The Power of the Market in Shaping a New Genomic Order, Goodenough-Chevening Conference, Goodenough-Chevening College, London.

Cooper, R. (1992) Formal Organization as Representation: Remote Control, Displacement and Abbreviation. In M. Reed and M. Hughes (Eds) *Rethinking Organization: New Directions in Organization Theory*, London: Sage. pp.254–72.

Cooper, R. (1997) The visibility of social systems. In K. Hetherington and R. Munro (Eds), *Ideas of Difference: Social Spaces and the Labour of Division*. Oxford: Blackwell/The Sociological Review. pp.32–41.

Cox, S.M. and Starzomski, R.C. (2004) Genes and Geneticization? The Social Construction of Autosomal Dominant Polycystic Kidney Disease. *New Genetics and Society*, 23 (2): 137–66.

Crawford, P. (2004) *Blood, Bodies and Families in Early Modern England*. Harlow, UK: Pearson Education.

Curtis, B. (2002) Foucault on Governmentality and Population: The Impossible Discovery. *Canadian Journal of Sociology*, 27 (4): 505–33.

Cussins, C. (1996) Ontological Choreography: Agency through Signification in Infertility Clinics. *Social Studies of Science*, 26 (3): 575–610.

Cussins, C. (1998) Ontological Choreography: Agency for Women in an Infertility Clinic. In M. Berg and A. Mol (Eds) *Differences in Medicine: Unravelling Practices, Techniques and Bodies*. Durham, NC and London: Duke University Press. pp.166–201.

D'Agincourt-Canning, L. (2001) Experiences of Genetic Risk: Disclosure and the Gendering of Responsibility. *Bioethics*, 15 (3): 231–47.

de Chadarevian, S. and Kamminga, H. (1998) *Introduction*. In de Chadarevian, S. and Kamminga, H. (Eds) *Molecularizing Biology and Medicine. New Practices and Alliances, 1910s–1970s*, Amsterdam: Harwood Academic Publishers. pp.1–15.

de Chadarevian, S. and Harmke, K. (Eds) (1998) *Molecularizing Biology and Medicine: New Practices and Alliances, 1910s–1970s.* Amsterdam: Harwood Academic Publishers.

Daly, K. (2004) *The Changing Culture of Parenting.* Virtual Library. The Vanier Institute of the Family. Ottawa, Ontario: The Vanier Institute. http://30645.vws.magma.ca/node/400 (Accessed September 2011).

Delaney, C. (2000) *Abraham on Trial: The Social Legacy of Biblical Myth.* Princeton: Princeton University Press.

Deleuze, G. (1988) *Foucault,* London: Athlone.

Deleuze, G. (1997) *Essays Critical and Clinical.* Translated by Daniel Smith and Michael A. Greco. New York: W.W. Norton & Company, Incorporated.

Deleuze, G. and Guattari, F. (1987) *A Thousand Plateaus. Capitalism and Schizophrenia.* Translated by Brian Massumi. Minneapolis: University of Minnesota Press.

Deleuze, G. and Parnet, F. (1987) *Dialogues 11.* Translated by Hugh Tomlinson and Barbara Habberjam. New York: Columbia University Press.

Delvecchio Good, M-J. (2001) The Biotechnical Embrace. *Culture, Medicine, and Psychiatry,* 25: 395–410.

Derbyshire, P. (1994) *Living with a Sick Child in Hospital.* Cheltenham, Glos: Nelson Thorne.

Derbyshire, S. (2012) The Problem of Infant Neurodeterminism. Paper presented at Medical and Scientific Understandings of Childhood Difference: Framings, Representations and Imaginaries, Policy, Ethics and Life Sciences Research Centre, Newcastle University, February 2012, Great North Museum, Newcastle upon Tyne.

Derrida, J. (1977) *Of Grammatology.* Baltimore, MD: Johns Hopkins University Press.

Derrida, J. (1978) *Writing and Difference.* Translated Alan Bass. London and New York: Routledge.

Didi-Huberman, G. (2004) *Invention of Hysteria. Charcot and the Photographic Iconography of the Salpetriere.* Translated by Alisa Hartz. Cambridge, Mass.: MIT Press.

Dikötter, F. (1998) *Imperfect Conceptions: Medical Knowledge, Birth Defects and Eugenics in China.* Columbia: Columbia University Press.

Dillon, M. and Reid, J. (2001) Global Liberal Governance: Biopolitics, Security and War. *Millennium: Journal of International Studies,* 30 (1): 41–66.

Dingwall, R. and Murray, T. (1983) Categorisation in Accident and Emergency Departments: 'Good' Patients, 'Bad' Patients and 'Children'. *Sociology of Health and Illness,* 5 (2): 127–48.

DOH (Department of Health) (2004) Patient and Public Involvement in Health: The Evidence for Policy Implementation. http://www.dh.gov.uk/PublicationsAndStatistics/Publications/PublicationsPolicyAndGuidance/PublicationsPolicyAndGuidance (Accessed September 2011).

Donnai, D. (2008) Basic Concepts in Dysmorphology and Syndrome Classification. http://eurogene.open.ac.uk/content/basic-concepts-dysmorphology-and-syndrome-classification-2008-0 (Accessed March 2011).

Douglas, M. (1966) *Purity and Danger.* Harmondsworth, Middlesex: Penguin.

Douglas, M. (1975) *Implicit Meanings: Essays in Anthropology.* London; New York: Routledge.

Douglas, M. (2003 [1970]) *Natural Symbols: Explorations in Cosmology.* London: Routledge.

Dunn, L.C. (1962) Cross Currents in the History of Human Genetics. *The American Journal of Human Genetics,* 14 (1): 1–13.

Duster, T. (1990) *Backdoor to Eugenics*. New York: Routledge.

Edwards, J. and Strathern, M. (2000) Including Our Own. In J. Carsten (Ed.) *Cultures of Relatedness: New Approaches to the Study of Kinship*. Cambridge: Cambridge University Press. pp.149–66.

Egorova, Y., Edgar, A. and Pattison, S. (2006) The Meanings of Genetics: Accounts of Biotechnology in the Work of Habermas, Derrida and Baudrillard. *International Journal of the Humanities*, 3 (2): 97–104.

Ettore, E. (2002) *Reproductive Genetics, Gender and the Body*. London: Routledge.

Fairclough, C. and Lee, E. (2010) Introduction: 'Changing Parenting Culture'. *Sociological Research Online*, 15 (4), http://www.socresonline.org.uk/15/4/1.html (Accessed May 2012).

Featherstone, K. and Atkinson, P. (2011) *Creating Conditions: the Making and Re-Making of a Genetic Syndrome*. London: Routledge.

Featherstone, K., Atkinson, P., Bharadwaj, A. and Clarke, A. (2006) *Risky Relations: Family, Kinship and the New Genetics*. Oxford: Berg.

Featherstone, K., Gregory, M. and Atkinson, P. (2006) The moral and sentimental work of the clinic: the case of dysmorphology. In P. Atkinson, P. Glasner and H. Greenslade (Eds) *New Genetics, New Identities*. London: Routledge.

Featherstone, K., Latimer, J., Atkinson, P., Pilz, D. and Clarke, A. (2005) Dysmorphology and the Spectacle of the Clinic. *Sociology of Health and Illness*, 27 (5): 551–74.

Featherstone, M. (2001) The Body in Consumer Culture. In M. Purdy and D. Banks (Eds) *The Sociology and Politics of Health: A Reader*. London: Routledge. pp.228–36.

Fernandez, J. (1986) *Persuasions and Performances: The Play of Tropes in Culture*. Bloomington: Indiana University Press.

Finkler, K. (2000) *Experiencing the New Genetics*. Philadelphia: University of Pennsylvania Press.

Fischer, M.M.J. (2005) Technoscientific Infrastructures and Emergent Forms of Life: A Commentary. *American Anthropologist*, 107 (1): 55–61.

Fleck, L. (1979) *The Genesis and Development of a Scientific Fact*. Chicago: University of Chicago Press.

Flower, M.J. and Heath, D. (1993) Micro-Anatomo Politics: Mapping the Human Genome Project. *Culture, Medicine and Psychiatry*, 17 (1): 27–41.

Foucault, M. (1979a) My Body, This Paper, This Fire. *Oxford Literary Review*, 4 (1): 9–28.

Foucault, M. (1979b) The life of infamous men. In M. Morris and P. Patton (Eds). Translated by Paul Foss and Meaghan Morris. *Michel Foucault: Power, Truth, Strategy*. Sydney: Feral Publications. pp.78–9.

Foucault, M. (1983) *This is Not a Pipe*. Berkely, California: University of California Press.

Foucault, M. (1991) Politics and the Study of Discourse. In G. Burchell, C. Gordon and P. Miller. *The Foucault Effect: Studies in Governmentality*. London: Harvester Wheatsheaf. pp.87–104.

Foucault, M. (1994 [1970]) *The Order of Things: An Archaeology of the Human Sciences*. New York: Vintage Books.

Foucault, M. (1995 [1977]) *Discipline & Punish: The Birth of the Prison*. Translated by Alan Sheridan. NY: Vintage Books.

Foucault, M. (1996 [1980]) 'The Masked Philosopher'. In S. Lotringer (Ed.) *Foucault Live (Interviews, 1961–1984)*. Translated by Lysa Hochroth and John Johnston. 2nd edition. New York: Semiotext(e).

Foucault, M. (2000a [1980]) The Politics of Health in the Eighteenth Century. *Power: Essential Works of Foucault, 1954–1984*, Volume III. Harmondsworth, UK: Penguin. pp.90–105.

Foucault, M. (2000b [1974]) The Birth of Social Medicine. *Power: Essential Works of Foucault, 1954–1984*, Volume III. pp.134–56.

Foucault, M. (2003a [1973]) *The Birth of the Clinic. An Archeology of Medical Perception.* London: Routledge.

Foucault, M. (2003b) Abnormal. *Lectures at the College de France, 1974–75*. New York: Picador.

Foucault, M. (2004 [1974]) The Crisis of Medicine or the Crisis of Antimedicine? Translated by Edgar C. Knowlton, Jr., William J. King and Clare O'Farrell. *Foucault Studies*, 1: 5–19.

Fox, N. (2012) *The Body*. Cambridge: Polity Press.

Fox, N.J., Ward, K.J. and O'Rourke, A.J. (2005) The 'Expert Patient': Empowerment or Medical Dominance? The Case of Weight Loss, Pharmaceutical Drugs and the Internet. *Social Science and Medicine*, 60 (6): 1299–309.

Frank, A.W. (1990) Bringing Bodies Back in: a Decade Review. *Theory, Culture and Society*, 7: 131–62.

Frankenberg, R. (1986) Sickness as Cultural Performance: Drama, Trajectory and Pilgrimage. Root Metaphors and the Making of Social Disease. *International Journal of Health Services*, 16 (4): 603–26.

Franklin, S. (2001) Biologization Revisited: Kinship Theory in the Context of the New Biologies. In S. Franklin and S. McKinnon (Eds) *Relative Values: Reconfiguring Kinship Studies*. Durham, NC: Duke University Press. pp.302–28.

Fraser, M. and Greco, M. (2005) Introduction. In M. Fraser and M. Greco (Eds) *The Body: A Reader*. London: Routledge. pp.1–42.

Freidson, E. (1988 [1970]) *Profession of Medicine: A Study of the Sociology of Applied Knowledge*. Chicago: University of Chicago Press.

Fujimura, J. (1996) *Crafting Science: A Sociohistory of the Quest for the Genetics of Cancer*. Cambridge, MA: Harvard University Press.

Fuller, S. (2007) *New Frontiers in Science and Technology Studies*. Cambridge, UK: Polity Press.

Gabe J., Bury M. and Elston M.A. (2004) *Key Concepts in Medical Sociology*. London: Sage.

Galison, P. (1994) *Big Science: The Growth of Large Scale Research*. Stanford, CA: Stanford University Press.

Galton, F. (1904) Eugenics: Its Definition, Scope, and Aims. *The American Journal of Sociology*, X (1), http://galton.org/essays/1900-1911/galton-1904-am-journ-soc-eugen-ics-scope-aims.htm (Accessed March 2012).

Garfinkel, H. (1967) *Studies in Ethnomethodology*. Englewood Cliffs, NJ: Prentice-Hall.

Gaudillière, J-P. (1992) Biochimistes et biomédecine dans l'après-guerre: deux itineraires entre laboratoire et hôpital. *Sciences Sociales et Santé*, 10: 107–47.

Gaudillière, J-P. (1993) Oncogenes as Metaphors for Human Cancer: Articulating Laboratory Practices and Medical Demands. In I. Löwy (Ed.) *Medicine and Change*. Paris: John Libbey. pp.212–448.

Gaudillière, J-P. (2002) *Inventer la biomédecine: La France, l'Amerique et la Production des Savoirs du Vivant Après 1945*. Paris: La Découverte.

Gaudillière, J-P. (2005) The Molecularization of Cancer Etiology in the Postwar United States: Instruments, Politics and Management. In S. de Chadarevian and H. Kamminga (Eds) *Molecularizing Biology and Medicine: New Practices and Alliances, 1910s–1970s*, Amsterdam: Harwood Academic Publishers. pp.129–59.

Gaudillière, J-P. and Löwy, I. (Eds) (1998) *Invisible Industrialists: Manufactures and the Production of Scientific Knowledge*. London: Macmillan.

Geertz, C. (1973) *The Interpretation of Cultures: Selected Essays*. London: Fontana Press.

Genetic Diseases (undated) http://www.genetic-diseases.net/down-syndrome/ (Accessed October 2011).

Gibbon, S. (2002) Re-examining Geneticization: Family Trees in Breast Cancer Genetics. *Science as Culture*, 11 (4): 429–57.

Gilman, S.L. (1988) *Disease and Representation: Images of Illness from Madness to AIDS*. Ithaca, New York: Cornell University Press.

Ginsburg, F. and Rapp, R. (1991) The Politics of Reproduction. *Annual Review of Anthropology*, 20: 311–43.

Goffman, E. (1963) *Stigma: Notes on the Management of Spoiled Identity*. New York: Simon and Schuster, Inc.

Goffman, E. (1980 [1968]) *The Presentation of Self in Everyday Life*. Harmondsworth, UK: Penguin Books.

Goffman, E. (1999 [1955]) *On Face-Work: An Analysis of Ritual Elements in Social Interaction*. In A. Jaworski and N. Coupland (Eds) *The Discourse Reader*. London: Routledge. pp.306–20.

Goffman, E. (2005 [1967]) *Interaction Ritual: Essays in Face-to-Face Behaviour*. Bunswick, NJ: Transaction Books.

Good, B. (1997) *Medicine, Rationality and Experience. An Anthropological Perspective*. Cambridge: Cambridge University Press.

Grace, V. (2003) Medical visualisation: Ontological politics and paradoxes. In V. Grace, H. Worth and L. Simmons (Eds) *Baudrillard West of the Dateline*. Palmerston North: Dunmore Press. pp.189–206.

Gray, D.E. (2002) 'Everybody just freezes. Everybody is just embarrassed': felt and enacted stigma among parents of children with high functioning autism. *Sociology of Health & Illness*, 24 (6): 734–49.

Greco, M. (2009) On the art of life: a vitalist reading of medical humanities. In J. Latimer and M. Schillmeier (Eds) *Un/knowing Bodies*. Sociological Review Monograph 56 (s2). Oxford: Wiley-Blackwell. pp.23–45.

Green, S.E. (2009) "What do you mean 'what's wrong with her?'": stigma and the lives of families of children with disabilities. *Social Science & Medicine*, 57 (8): 1361–74.

Grosz, E. (1993) Bodies and Knowledges: Feminism and the Crisis of Reason. In L. Alcoff and E. Potter (Eds) *Feminist Epistemologies*. New York/London: Routledge. pp.187–216.

Habermas, J. (2003) *The Future of Human Nature*. Translated by Hella Beister and William Rehg. Cambridge: Polity Press.

Hacking, I. (1983) *Representing and Intervening: Introductory Topics in the Philosophy of Natural Science*. Cambridge: Cambridge University Press.

Hacking, I. (1986) 'Making People Up'. In T.C. Heller, D.E. Wellbery and M. Sosna (Eds) *Reconstructing Individualism: Autonomy, Individuality and the Self in Western Thought*. Stanford, CA: Stanford University Press.

Hacking, I. (2006) Genetics, biosocial groups & the future of identity. *Daedalus*, 135 (4): 81–95.

Halfmann, D. (2011) Recognizing Medicalization and Demedicalization: Discourses, Practices and Identities, *Health*, 3 May, http://hea.sagepub.com/content/early/2011/05/07/1363459311403947 (Accessed January 2012).

Haraway, D.J. (1989) The Biopolitics of Postmodern Bodies: Determinations of Self in Immune System Discourse. *Differences: A Journal of Feminist Cultural Studies*, 1 (1): 3–43.

Haraway, D. (1991) *Simians, Cyborgs and Women: The Reinvention of Nature*. New York: Routledge.

Haraway, D. (2007) *When Species Meet*. Minneapolis: University of Minnesota Press.

Harper, P. (2006) *First Years of Human Chromosomes*. Bloxham, Oxfordshire: Scion Press.

Harper, P. (2008) *A Short History of Medical Genetics*. Oxford: Oxford University Press.

Harper, P. (Ed.) (2004) *Landmarks in Medical Genetics: A Collection of Classic Papers with Commentaries*. Oxford: Oxford University Press.

Hayles K. (1999) *How We Became Posthuman: Virtual Bodies in Cybernetics, Literature and Informatics*. Chicago: The University of Chicago Press.

Heath, C. and vom Lehn, D. (2008) Museums Configuring 'Interactivity': Enhancing Engagement in Science Centres and Museums. *Social Studies of Science*, 38 (1): 63–91.

Hedgecoe, A. (1998) Geneticization, medicalization and polemics. *Medicine, Health Care and Philosophy*, 1 (3): 235–43.

Hedgecoe, A. (2002) Reinventing Diabetes: Classification, Division, and the Geneticization of Disease. *New Genetics and Society*, 21 (1): 7–27.

Hedgecoe, A. (2003) Expansion and Uncertainty: Cystic Fibrosis, Classification and Genetics. *Sociology of Health and Illness*, 25 (1): 50–70.

Hedgecoe, A. (2004a) A Reply to Ann Kerr. *Sociology of Health and Illness*, 26 (1): 107–9.

Hedgecoe, A. (2004b) *The Politics of Personalized Medicine: Pharmacogenetics in the Clinic*. Cambridge: Cambridge University Press.

Hedgecoe, A. and Tutton, R. (2002) Guest Editorial: Genetics in Society/Society in Genetics. *Science as Culture*, 11 (4): 421–8.

Hetherington, K. (2011) Foucault, the museum and the diagram. *Sociological Review*, 59 (3): 457–75.

Hewitt, M. (1983) Biopolitics and Social Policy: Foucault's Account of Welfare. *Theory, Culture and Society*, 2 (1): 67–84.

Hillman, A., Latimer, J. and White, P. (2010) Accessing Care: Technology and the Management of the Clinic. In M. Schillmeier and M. Domenech (Eds) *New Technologies and Emerging Spaces of Care*. Farnham, Surrey: Ashgate. pp.197–220.

Hogle, L.F. (1995) Standardization Across Non-Standard Domains: The case of organ procurement. *Science, Technology and Human Values*, 20 (4): 482–500.

Howell, S. (2006) *The Kinning of Foreigners: Transnational Adoption in a Global Perspective*. Oxford: Berghahn Books.

Human Genetics Commission (2004) *Choosing the Future: Genetics and Reproductive Decision-Making*. London: Department of Health.

Human Genetics Commission (2006) *Making Babies: reproductive decisions and genetic technologies*, http://www.HGC.Gov.UK (Accessed March 2007).

Illich, I. (1976) *Medical Nemesis: The Expropriation of Health*. New York: Pantheon Books.

Ivens, A., Moore, G. and Williamson, R. (1988) Molecular Approaches to Dysmorphology. *Journal of Medical Genetics*, 25: 473–79.

Jamous, H. and Peloille, B. (1970) Professions of Self-Perpetuating System? In J.A. Jackson (Ed.) *Professions and Professionalisation*. Cambridge: Cambridge University Press. pp.109–52.

Jeffery, R. (1979) Normal Rubbish: Deviant Patients in Casualty Departments. *Sociology of Health and Illness*, 1 (1): 91–107.

Jordonova, L. (2000) *Defining Features: Scientific and Medical Portraits 1660–2000*. London: Reaktion Books/National Portrait Gallery.

Jordonova, L. (2003) Portraits, People and Things: Richard Mead and Medical Identity. *History of Science* (special issue in memory of Roy Porter), 61: 293–313.

Kaplan, J.M. (2000) *The Limits and Lies of Human Genetic Research. Dangers for Social Policy*. New York/London: Routledge.

Kara, B., Kayserili, H., Imer, M., Çashkan, M. and Özmen, M. (2006) Quadrigeminal Cistern Arachnoid Cyst in a Patient With Kabuki Syndrome. *Pediatric Neurology*, 34 (6): 478–80.

Kass, L.R. (2002) *Life, Liberty, and the Defense of Dignity: The Challenge for Bioethics*. San Francisco: Encounter Books.

Kaufman, S. (1994) Old Age, Disease, and the Discourse on Risk: Geriatric Assessment in U.S. Health Care. *Medical Anthropology Quarterly*, 8 (4): 430–47.

Kaushik, S.R. (2006) *Biocapital: The Constitution of Postgenomic Life*. Durham, NC: Duke University Press.

Keating, P. and Cambrosio, A. (2003) *Biomedical Platforms: Realigning the Normal and the Pathological in Late-Twentieth-Century Medicine*. Cambridge, MA: MIT Press.

Kelly, S.E. (2006) From scraps and fragments to whole organisms: Molecular biology, clinical research and post genomic bodies. In P. Atkinson and P. Glaser (Eds) *New Genetics, New Identities*. London: Routledge. pp.44–60.

Kemp M. and Wallace M. (2000) *Spectacular Bodies. The Art and Science of the Human Body from the Renaissance to Now*, London: Hayward Gallery and Berkley: University of California Press.

Kerr, A. (2000) (Re)constructing Genetic Disease: The Clinical Continuum Between Cystic Fibrosis and Male Infertility. *Social Studies of Science*, 30 (6): 847–94.

Kerr, A. (2004a) *Genetics and Society: A Sociology of Disease*. London: Routledge.

Kerr, A. (2004b) Giving up on Geneticization: A comment on Hedgecoe's 'Expansion and uncertainty: cystic fibrosis, classification and genetics'. *Sociology of Health and Illness*, 26 (1): 102–6.

King, L.S. (1982) *Medical Thinking: A Historical Perspective*. Princeton NJ: Princeton University Press.

Kinmonth, A.L. (1998) The New Genetics Implications for Clinical Services in Britain and the United States. *British Medical Journal*, 7: 316 (7133): 767–70.

Konrad, M. (2005) *Narrating the New Predictive Genetics: Ethics, Ethnography and Science*. Cambridge: Cambridge University Press.

Korf, B.R. (2002) Genetics in Medical Practice. *Genetics In Medicine*, 4 (6): 135–45.

Kuhn, T.S. (1970) *The Structure of Scientific Revolutions*. Chicago: University of Chicago Press.

Kukla, R. (2008) Measuring Motherhood. *International Journal of Feminist Bioethics*, 1 (1): 67–90.

Kundera, M. (1996) *Slowness*. London: Faber and Faber.

Lambert, H. and MacDonald, M. (2009) Introduction. In H. Lambert and M. MacDonald (Eds) *Social Bodies*. New York and Oxford: Berghahn Books. pp.1–16.

Lange, L. (2003) Woman is not a Rational Animal: On Aristotle's Biology of Reproduction. In S. Harding and M.B. Hintikka (Eds) *Discovering Reality. Feminist Perspectives on Epistemology, Metaphysics, Methodology, and Philosophy of Science*. 2nd Edition. Dordrecht, NL: Kluewer Academic Publishers. pp.1–15.

Latimer, J. (1997) Giving Patients a Future: The Constituting of Classes in an Acute Medical Unit. *Sociology of Health and Illness*, 19 (2): 160–85.

Latimer, J. (1999) The Dark at the Bottom of the Stair: Participation and performance of older people in hospital. *Medical Anthropology Quarterly*, 13 (2): 186–213.

Latimer, J. (2000) Socialising Disease: Medical Categories and Inclusion of the Aged. *The Sociological Review*, 48 (3): 383–407.

Latimer, J. (2004) Commanding Materials: (Re)Legitimating Authority in the Context of Multi-Disciplinary Work. *Sociology*, 38 (4): 757–75.

Latimer, J. (2007a) Diagnosis, Dysmorphology and the Family: Knowledge, Motility, Choice. *Medical Anthropology*, 26: 53–94.

Latimer, J. (2007b) Becoming In-formed: Genetic Counselling, Ambiguity and Choice. Special Issue on The Meaning of Genetics and Conceptions of Personhood. *Health Care Analysis*, 15 (2): 107–21.

Latimer, J. (2009a) Introduction: Body, Knowledge, World. In J. Latimer and M. Schillmeier (Eds) *Un/knowing Bodies*, Sociological Review Monograph Series. Sociological Review Online Special Issue: vol. 56, monograph 2, pp.1–22. Oxford: Wiley.

Latimer, J. (2009b) Unsettling Bodies: Frida Kahlo's Self-Portraits and Dividuality. In J. Latimer and M. Schillmeier (Eds) *Un/knowing Bodies*, Sociological Review Monograph Series. Sociological Review Online Special Issue: vol. 56, monograph 2, pp.46–62. Oxford: Wiley.

Latimer, J. (2011) Home, Care and Frail Older People: Relational extension & the art of dwelling. In C. Ceci, M.E. Purkis and K. Björnsdóttir (Eds) *Homecare: International and Comparative Perspectives*. London: Routledge.

Latimer, J. (2013) Rewriting bodies, portraiting persons? The gene, the clinic and the (post) human. *Body & Society*, On-line First, bod.sagepub.com/content/early/recent.

Latimer, J., Featherstone, K., Atkinson, P., Clarke, A., Pilz, D. and Shaw, A. (2006) Rebirthing the clinic: the interaction of clinical judgment and genetic technology in the production of medical science. *Science, Technology and Human Values*, 31 (5): 599–630.

Latimer, J. and Munro, R. (2006) Driving the Social. In S. Bohm, C. Jones and M. Pattison (Eds) *Against Automobility*. Sociological Review Monograph. 54, Issue Supplement s1, October: 32–55. Oxford: Blackwell.

Latimer, J. and Skeggs, B. (2011) The Politics of Imagination: Keeping Open & Critical. *The Sociological Review*, 59 (3): 493–410.

Latour, B. (1986) The Powers of Association. In J. Law (Ed.) *Power, Action and Belief: a New Sociology of Knowledge?* London, Boston and Henley: Routledge and Kegan Paul. pp.264–80.

Latour, B. (1987) *Science in Action*. Milton Keynes: Open University Press.

Latour, B. (1988) *The Pasteurization of France*. Cambridge, MA: MIT University Press.

Latour, B. (1989) Clothing the Naked Truth. In H. Lawson and L. Appignanesi (Eds) *Dismantling Truth. Reality in the Post-Modern World*. London: Weidenfeld and Nicolson. pp.145–65.

Latour, B. (1993 [1991]) *We Have Never Been Modern*. Translated by Catherine Porter. Cambridge, MA: Harvard University Press.

Latour, B. (2004) How to Talk About the Body? The Normative Dimension of Science Studies. *Body & Society*, 10: 205–29.

Law, J. (1992) Notes on the Theory of Actor-Network: Ordering, Strategy, and Heterogeneity. *Systems Practice*, 5, 379–93.

Leder, D. (1990) *The Absent Body*. Chicago: University of Chicago.

Lee, E. (2012) Prejudice Masquerading as Research: Brain Science and British Social Policy. Paper Presentation, *Medical and Scientific Understandings of Childhood Difference: Framings, Representations and Imaginaries*, Policy, Ethics and Life

Sciences Research Centre, Newcastle University, February 2012, Great North Museum, Newcastle upon Tyne.

Lee, N.M. (1998) Towards an Immature Sociology. *The Sociological Review*, 46 (3): 458–82.

Lee, N.M. (2001) *Childhood and Society: growing up in an age of uncertainty*. Buckingham: Open University Press.

Lee, N.M. (2009) Researching children's diets in England: critical methods in a consumer society. *Qualitative Research in Psychology*, 6 (1–2): 88–104.

Levy, R., Widmer, E. and Kellerhals, J. (2002) Modern Family or Modernized Family Traditionalism?: Master Status and the Gender Order in Switzerland. *Electronic Journal of Sociology*, 6 (4).

Lisle, L. (1999) *Without Child: Challenging the Stigma of Childlessness*. London: Routledge.

Lock, M. and Kaufert, P. (1998) *Pragmatic Women and Body Politics*. Cambridge: Cambridge University Press.

Loeys, B.L. *et al.* (2010) The revised Ghent nosology for the Marfan syndrome. *Journal of Medical Genetics*, 47 (7): 476–85.

Lombroso, C. with Lombroso-Ferrero, G. (1972 [(1911]) *Criminal Man, According to the Classification of Cesare Lombroso*. New York: Putnam.

Loos, H.S., Wieczorek, D., Wurtz R.P., von der Malsburg, C. and Horsthemke B. (2003) Computer-Based Recognition of Dysmorphic Faces. *European Journal of Human Genetics*, 11: 555–60.

Long, J. (1992) Foucault's Clinic. *The Journal of Medical Humanities*, 13 (3): 119–38.

Löwy, I. (1996) *Between Bench and Bedside: Science, Healing and Interleukin-2 in a Cancer Ward*. Cambridge: Harvard University Press.

Lupton, D. (2005) *Limits to Medicine: Medical Nemesis. Journal of Health Services Research and Policy*, 10 (2): 122–3.

Lynch, M. (1985) Discipline and the Material Form of Images: An Analysis of Scientific Visibility. *Social Studies of Science*, 15 (1): 37–66.

Lyotard, J-F. (1984) *The Postmodern Condition. A Report on Knowledge*. Translated by Geoffrey Bennington and Brian Massumi. Manchester: Manchester University Press.

McLaughlin, J. and Clavering, E.K. (2011) Questions of kinship and inheritance in pediatric genetics: substance and responsibility. *New Genetics and Society*, 30 (4): 399–413.

Mahowald, M.B., Verp, M.S. and Anderson, R.R. (1998) Genetic Counselling: Clinical and Ethical Challenges. *Annual Review of Genetics*, 32: 547–59.

Martin, A. (2010) Microchimerism in the Mother(land): Blurring the Borders of Body and Nation. *Body & Society*, 16 (3): 23–50.

Martin, E. (1991) The Egg and the Sperm – How Science has Constructed a Romance Based on Stereotypical Male-Female Roles. *Signs*, 16 (3): 485–501.

Martin, E. (1998) Anthropology and the Cultural Study of Science. *Science, Technology and Human Values*, 23 (2): 24–44.

Martin, E. (2004) Talking Back to Neuro-reductionism. In H. Thomas and J. Ahmed, (Eds) *Cultural Bodies*. Oxford: Blackwell. pp.190–211.

Marx, K. (1991) *Capital*, vol. 3. Harmondsworth: Penguin.

Mathews, A. (1999) *Vienna Blood*. London: Vintage.

Mauss, M. (1973) Techniques of the body. *Economy and Society*, 2 (1): 70–88.

May, C. (1992) Individual care? Power and subjectivity in therapeutic relationships. *Sociology*, 26: 589–602.

McKusick, V.A. (1998 [1966]) *Mendelian Inheritance in Man. A Catalog of Human Genes and Genetic Disorders*, 12th Edn. Baltimore, MD: Johns Hopkins University Press.

Melley, T. (2002) A Terminal Case: William Burroughs and the Logic of Addiction. In M. Redfield and J. Farrell (Eds) *High Anxieties: Cultural Studies in Addiction*. Berkeley: University of California Press. pp.38–60.

Miller, F. (1999) An Interview with Abby Lippman on the New Genetics. Canadian Women's Health Network. Network 2(2). http://www.cwhn.ca/networkreseau/2-2/ interview.html

Mol, A-M. (2000) Pathology and the Clinic: an Ethnographic Presentation of Two Atheroscleroses. In M. Lock, A. Young and A. Cambrosio (Eds) *Living and Working with the New Medical Technologies: Intersections of Inquiry*. Cambridge, UK: Cambridge University Press. pp.82–102.

Mol, A-M. (2002) *The Body Multiple: Ontology in Medical Practice*. Durham, North Carolina: Duke University Press.

Moreira, T. (2004) Self, Agency and Surgery: Detachment. *Sociology of Health and Illness*, 26 (1): pp.1–18.

Morris, C.A. (2006) Dysmorphology, Genetics, and Natural History of Williams-Beuren Syndrome: An Overview. In C.A. Morris, P.P. Wang and H. Lenhoff (Eds) *Williams-Beuren Syndrome: Research and Clinical Perspectives*. Baltimore, MD: Johns Hopkins University Press. pp.3–18.

Moss, P. and Teghtsoonian, K. (2008) Power and Illness: Authority, Bodies, Context. In P. Moss and K. Teghtsoonian (Eds) *Contesting Illness: Process and Practices*. Toronto: Toronto University Press. pp.3–27.

Munro, R. (1995) Governing the New Province of Quality: Autonomy, Accounting and the Dissemination of Accountability. In A. Wilkinson and H. Willmott (Eds) *Making Quality Critical*. London: Routledge. pp.127–55.

Munro, R. (1996) The Consumption View of Self: Extension, Exchange and Identity. In S. Edgell, K. Hetherington and A. Warde (Eds) *Consumption Matters*. Sociological Review Monograph. Oxford: Blackwell. pp. 248–73.

Munro, R. (1999a) Power and Discretion: membership work in the time of technology. *Organization*, 6 (3): 429–50.

Munro, R. (1999b) Managing by Ambiguity: An Archeology of the Social in the Absence of Management Accounting. *Critical Perspectives on Accounting*, 6 (4): 433–82.

Munro, R. (2003) Structure: Disorganization. In R. Westwood and S. Clegg (Eds) *Point/Counterpoint: Central Debates in Organisation Theory*. Oxford: Blackwell. pp.283–97.

Munro, R. (2005) Partial Organization: Marilyn Strathern and the Elicitation of Relations. In C. Jones and R. Munro (Eds) *Contemporary Organization Theory*. Oxford: Blackwell. pp.245–66.

Munro, R. and Belova, O. (2008) The body in time: knowing bodies and the 'interruption' of narrative. In J. Latimer and M. Schillmeier (Eds) *Un/knowing Bodies*, Sociological Review Online Special Issue: vol. 56, monograph 2, pp.85–99.

Munro, R. and Mouritsen, J. (Eds) (1996) *Accountability: Power, Ethos and the Technologies of Managing*. London: International Thomson Business Press.

Myers, G. (1990) The Double Helix as Icon. *Science as Culture*, 1 (9): 49–72.

National Institute of Neurological Disorders and Stroke (undated) Coffin Lowry Syndrome Information Page. http://www.ninds.nih.gov/disorders/coffin_lowry/coffin_lowry.htm (Accessed July 2005).

Navarro, V. (1988) Professional Dominance or Proletarianization?: Neither. *The Milbank Quarterly*. The Changing Character of the Medical Profession, 66 (2): 57–75.

Newman, K. (1996) *Fetal Positions: Individualism, Science, Visuality (Writing Science)*. Stanford, CA: Stanford University Press.

Novas, C. and Rose, N. (2000) Genetic Risk and the birth of the somatic individual. *Economy and Society*, 29 (4) November: 485–513.

NSF (National Science Foundation) (2010) About the National Science Foundation http://www.nsf.gov/about/ (Accessed December 2012).

Nukaga, Y. and Cambrosio, A. (1997) Medical Pedigrees and the Visual Production of Family Disease in Canadian and Japanese Genetic Counselling Practice. In M.A. Elston (Ed) *The Sociology of Medical Science and Technology*. Oxford: Blackwell. pp.29–55.

Nye, R. (2003) The Evolution of the Concept of Medicalization in the Late Twentieth Century. *Journal of History of the Behavioral Sciences*, 39 (2): 115–29.

OECD. Health Data. (2004) Total Expenditure as % of GDP by Country, http://www.NationMaster.com/red/graph/hea_tot_exp_as_of_gdp-health-total-expenditure-gdp&b_printable=1 (Accessed May 2010).

O'Farrell, C. (2007) Key Concepts. http://www.michel-foucault.com/concepts/index.html (Accessed March 2012).

Okely, J. (1999) Love, Care and Diagnosis. In T. Kohn and R. McKechnie (Eds) *Extending the Boundaries of Care: Medical Ethics and Caring Practices*. Oxford: Berg. pp.19–48.

Olshansky, S.J. and Carnes, B.A. (2001) The Quest for Immortality. *Science at the Frontiers of Ageing*. New York: W.W. Norton.

Osbourne, T. (1992) Medicine and Epistemology: Michel Foucault and the Liberality of Clinical Reason. *History of the Human Sciences*, 5 (2): 63–93.

Oudshoorn, N. (1996) A Natural Order of Things? Reproductive Science and the Politics of Othering. In G. Robertson, M. Mash, L. Tickner, J. Bird, B. Curtis and T. Putnam (Eds) *FutureNatural: Nature, Science, Culture*. New York: Routledge. pp.121–32.

Pálsson, G. (2007) *Anthropology and the New Genetics*. Cambridge, UK: Cambridge University Press.

Pandora's Box (undated) http://www.consultsos.com/pandora/fescupht.htm. (Accessed December 2011).

Papadopoulos, D. (2011) The imaginary of plasticity: Neural embodiment, epigenetics and ecomorphs. *Sociological Review*, 59 (3): 432–56.

Parker, M. (2000) Public Deliberation and Private Choice in Genetics and Reproduction. *Journal of Medical Ethics*, 26 (3): 160–5.

Parsons, E., Clarke A. and Bradley D.M. (2003) Implications of carrier identification in newborn screening for cystic fibrosis. *Archives of Disease in Childhood: Fetal & Neonatal*, 88: F467–F471.

Parsons, T. (1964 [1951]) *Social System*. Chicago: Free Press.

Parsons, T. (1991 [1951]) *Social System*. London: Routledge and Kegan Paul Ltd.

Pinkowski, J. (2004) The Alchemist's Lab. *Archeology*, 57 (6): 26–9.

Pray, L. (2008) Embryo Screening and the Ethics of Human Genetic Engineering. *Nature Education*, 1 (1), http://www.nature.com/scitable/topicpage/embryo-screening-and-the-ethics-of-60561 (Accessed February 2011).

President's Council on Bioethics (2003a) *Beyond Therapy: Biotechnology and the Pursuit of Happiness* (Report). The President's Council on Bioethics, Washington, DC,

October, http://bioethics.georgetown.edu/pcbe/reports/beyondtherapy/index.html (Accessed May 2009).

President's Council on Bioethics (2003b) *Being Human: Readings from the President's Council on Bioethics*. The President's Council on Bioethics, Washington, DC, December, http://bioethics.georgetown.edu/pcbe/bookshelf/index.html.

Purkis, M.E. (2002) Governing the health of populations: The child, the clinic and the 'conversation'. In V. Hayes and L. Young (Eds) *Transforming Health Promotion Practice: Concepts, Issues, and Applications*. F.A. Davis: Philadelphia. pp.190–206.

Purkis, M.E. (2003) Moving Nursing Practice: Integrating Theory and Method. In J. Latimer (Ed.) *Advanced Qualitative Research for Nursing*. Oxford: Blackwell. pp.32–50.

Rabeharisoa V. and Callon M. (2004) Patients and scientists in French muscular dystrophy research. In S. Jasanoff (Ed.) *States of Knowledge: The co-production of science and social order*. London: Routledge. pp.142–60.

Rabinow, P. (1992) Artificiality and Enlightenment: From Sociobiology to Biosociality. In J. Crary and S. Kwinter (Eds) *Incorporations*. New York: Urzone. pp.91–126.

Rabinow, P. (1996) *Making PCR, A Story of Biotechnology*. Chicago: University of Chicago Press.

Rabinow, P. (2000) Epochs, Presents, Events. In M. Lock, A. Young and A. Cambrosio (Eds) *Living and Working with the New Medical Technologies: Intersections of Inquiry*. Cambridge: Cambridge University Press. pp.31–48.

Rabinow, P. and Rose, N. (2006) Thoughts on the Concept of Biopower Today. *BioSocieties*, 1: 195–217.

Rajan, K.S. (2006) *BioCapital: The Constitution of PostGenomic Life*. Durham and London: Duke University Press.

Rao, R. (1996) Assisted Reproductive Technology and the Threat to the Traditional Family, 47 Hastings L.J. 951, http://faculty.law.miami.edu/mcoombs/documents/rao.doc (Accessed December 2011).

Reardon, W. and Donnai, D. (2007) Dysmorphology Demystified. *Archives of Diseases in Childhood: Fetal & Neonatal*. 92: F225–F229, http://fn.bmj.com/content/92/3/F225.extract (Accessed September 2011).

Regalado, M. and Halfon, N. (2001) Primary Care Services: Promoting Optimal Child Development From Birth to Age 3 Years. Review of the Literature. *Archives of Pediatrics & Adolescent Medicine*, 155: 1311–22.

Rheinberger, H-J. (1997) *Toward a History of Epistemic Things: Synthesizing Proteins in the Test Tube*. Stanford: Stanford University Press.

Rheinberger, H-J. (2000) Beyond Nature and Culture: Modes of Reasoning in the Age of Molecular Biology and Medicine. In M. Lock, A. Young and A. Cambrosio (Eds) *Living and Working with the New Medical Technologies: Intersections of Inquiry*. Cambridge, UK: Cambridge University Press. pp.19–30.

Richards, M. (2002) Future Bodies: Some History and Future Prospects for Human Genetic Selection. In A. Bainham, M. Richards and S. Day Sclater (Eds) *Body Lore and Laws*. Oxford and Portland, Oregon: Hart Publishing. pp.289–307.

Robertson, S.G. and Bankier, A. (1999) Sotos syndrome and cutis laxa. *Journal of Medical Genetics*, 36: 51–6.

Roeher Institute (2002) *The Construction of Disability and Risk in Genetic Counselling*. Ottawa: Status of Women.

Rose, N. (1999) *Powers of Freedom: Reframing Political Thought*. Cambridge: Cambridge University Press.

Rose, N. (2001) The Politics of Life Itself. *Theory, Culture & Society*, 18 (6): 1–30.

Rose, N. (2007a) Beyond medicalisation. *The Lancet*, 369 (9562): 700–2.

Rose, N. (2007b) *The Politics of Life Itself: Biomedicine, Power, and Subjectivity in the Twenty-First Century*. Princeton: Princeton University Press.

Rose, N. and Novas, C. (2005) Biological Citizens. In A. Ong and S.J. Collier (Eds) *Global Assemblages: Technology, Politics, and Ethics as Anthropological Problems*. Oxford: Blackwell. pp.439–63.

Rothman B.K. (2004) Motherhood Under Capitalism. In J.S. Taylor, L.L. Layne and D.F. Wozniak (Eds) *Consuming Motherhood*. New Brunswick, NJ: Rutgers University Press. pp.19–30.

Sarangi, S. and Clarke, A.J. (2002) Zones of Expertise and the Management of Uncertainty in Genetics Risk Communication. *Research on Language and Social Interaction*, 35 (2): 139–71.

Schilling, C. (2002) Culture, the 'Sick Role' and the Consumption of Health. *British Journal of Sociology*, 53 (4): 621–38.

Schneider, J.W. (2003 [1978]) Deviant Drinking as a Disease: Alchoholism as a Social Accomplishment. In Conrad, P. and Leiter, V. (Eds) *Health and Heath Care as Social Problems*. Lanham, Maryland: Rowman and Little. pp.9–23.

Seale, C., Pattison, S. and Davey, B. (Eds) (2001) *Medical Knowledge: Doubt and Certainty*. Buckingham; Philadelphia: Open University Press.

Sekula, A. (1986) The Body and the Archive. *October*, 39: 3-64.

Selicorni, A. *et al.* (2007) Mental Retardation in Paediatric Disease. In D. Riva, S. Bulgheroni and C. Pantaleoni (Eds) *Mental Retardation*. Montrouge, France: John Libby Eurotext. pp.49–62.

Shapin, S. (2000) Descartes the Doctor: Rationalism and its Therapies. *British Journal for the History of Science*, 33: 131–54.

Shapin, S. (2008) *The Scientific Life: A Moral History of a Late Modern Vocation*. Chicago: Chicago University Press.

Shaw, J. (2012) The Birth of the Clinic and the Advent of Reproduction: Pregnancy, Pathology and the Medical Gaze in Modernity. *Body & Society*, 18: 110–38.

Shaw, J. and Baker, M. (2004) Expert patient: dream or nightmare? *British Medical Journal*, 328: 723–4.

Shaw, A., Latimer, J., Atkinson, P. and Featherstone, K. (2003) Surveying Slides: Clinical Perception and Clinical Judgment in the Construction of a Genetic Diagnosis. *New Genetics and Society*, 22 (1): 3–19.

Silverman, D. (1987) *Communication and Medical Practice: Social relations in the clinic*, London: Sage.

Silverman, D., Hilliard, R., Baruch, G. and Shinebourne, E. (1984) Factors Influencing Parental Participation in a Paediatric Cardiology Outpatient Clinic. *International Journal of Cardiology*, 6 (6): 689–98.

Sinding, C. (1989) The History of Resistant Rickets: A Model for Understanding the Growth of Medical Knowledge. *Journal of the History of Biology*, 22 (3): 461–95.

Sinding, C. (1990) Basic Science and Clinical Research: The Development of the Concept of Organ Resistance to a Hormone. *Journal of the History of Medicine and Allied Sciences*, 45 (3): 198–232.

Sinding, C. (1991) *Le Clinicien et le Chercheur: De Grandes Maladies de Carence à la Médicine Moleculaire, 1880–1980*. Paris: Presses Universitaires de France.

Skeggs, B. (2004) *Class, Self, Culture*. London: Routledge.

Skeggs, B. (2010) Class, culture and morality: legacies and logics in the space for identification. In M. Wetherell and C.T. Mohanty (Eds) *The Sage Handbook of Identities*. London: Sage. pp.339–60.

Skeggs, B. (2011) Imagining Personhood Differently: Person Value and Autonomist Working-Class Value Practices. In J. Latimer and B. Skeggs (Eds) The Politics of Imagination Special Issue. *The Sociological Review*, 9 (3): 496–513.

Skeggs, B. and Wood, H. (2008) The Labour of Transformation and Circuits of Value 'around' Reality Television. *Continuum: Journal of Media & Cultural Studies*, 22 (4): 559–72.

Skirton, H. and Barr, O. (2007) Influences on Uptake of Antenatal Screening for Down Syndrome: a Review of the Literature. *Evidence Based Midwifery*, 5 (1): 4–9.

Smart, C. (2004) Retheorizing Families. *Sociology*, 38 (5): 1043–8.

Smyth, I. and Scambler, P. (2005) The genetics of Fraser syndrome and the blebs mouse mutants. *Human Molecular Genetics*, 14 (2): R269–R274.

Sointu, E. (2005) The Rise of an Ideal: Tracing Changing Discourses of Well-Being. *The Sociological Review*, 53 (2): 255–74.

Stanford Encyclopedia of Philosophy (2004) The Genotype/Phenotype Distinction. http:// plato.stanford.edu/entries/genotype-phenotype/ (Accessed May 2010).

Star, S.L. (1989) *Regions of the Mind: Brain Research and the Quest for Scientific Certainty*. Stanford, CA: Stanford University Press.

Star, S.L. and Griesemer, J.R. (1989) *Institutional Ecology, 'Translations' and Boundary Objects: Amateurs and Professionals in Berkeley's Museum of Vertebrate Zoology, 1907–39*. In M. Biagioli (Ed.) *The Science Studies Reader*. New York/London: Routledge. pp. 503–24.

Stewart, A. (2004) Assessing the Public's Views on Genetics and Reproductive Decision-Making. http://www.cambridgenetwork.co.uk/POOLED/ARTICLES/BF_NEWSART/ VIEW.ASP?Q=BF_NEWSART_110937 (Accessed December 2005).

Strathern, M. (1988) *The Gender of the Gift*. Berkley, CA: University of California Press.

Strathern, M. (1991) *Partial Connections*. Maryland: Rowman and Littlefield Publishers Inc.

Strathern, M. (1992a) *After Nature: English Kinship in the Late Twentieth Century*. Cambridge: Cambridge University Press.

Strathern, M. (1992b) Parts and wholes: Refiguring Relationships in a Postplural World. In A. Kuper (Ed.), *Conceptualising Society*. London: Routledge. pp.75–104.

Strathern, M. (1992c) *Reproducing the Future: Anthropology, Kinship and the New Reproductive Technologies*. Cambridge: Cambridge University Press.

Strathern, M. (1995) *The Relation. Issues in Complexity and Scale*. Cambridge, UK: Prickley Pear Press.

Strathern, M. (1996) Enabling Identity? Biology, Choice and the New Reproductive Technologies. In S. Hall and P. du Gay (Eds) *Questions of Cultural Identity*. London: Sage. pp.37–42.

Strathern, M. (1997) Gender, Division or Comparison? In K. Hetherington and R. Munro (Eds) *Ideas of Difference. Social Spaces and the Labour of Division*. Sociological Review Monograph, Oxford: Wiley-Blackwell. pp.42–63.

Strathern, M. (2004a) Commons and borderlands: Working papers on interdisciplinarity, accountability and the flow of knowledge. Wantage: Sean Kingston Publishing.

Strathern, M. (2004b) Social Property: An Interdisciplinary Experiment. *PoLAR: Political and Legal Anthropology Review*, 27 (1): 23–50.

Strathern, M. (2005) *Kinship, Law and the Unexpected: Relatives are Always a Surprise*. Cambridge: University of Cambridge Press.

Strathern, M. (2009) Using Bodies to Communicate. In H. Lambert and M. MacDonald (Eds) *Social Bodies*. Oxford: Berghahn Books. pp.148–70.

Sykes, K.M. (2005) *Arguing with Anthropology: An Introduction to Critical Theories of the Gift.* London: Routledge.

Tauber, A.I. (1996) The Molecularization of Immunology. In S. Sarkar (Ed.) *The Philosophy and History of Molecular Biology: New Perspectives.* Dordrecht: Kluwer Academic Publishers. pp.125–69.

Taussig, M.T. (1980) Reification and the Consciousness of the Patient. *Social Science & Medicine*, Part B: Medical Anthropology, 14 (1): 3–13. (http://www.sciencedirect.com/science/article/pii/0160798780900356)

ten Have, H.A.M.J. (2012) Geneticisation: Concept. In *eLS*. John Wiley & Sons Ltd, Chichester   http://onlinelibrary.wiley.com/doi/10.1002/9780470015902.a0005896.pub2/abstract (Accessed June 2012).

Thompson, C. (2005) *Making Parents: The Ontological Choreography of Reproductive Technologies.* Cambridge, MA: MIT Press.

Thompson, D.W. (2000 [1961]) *On Growth and Form.* Cambridge, UK: Cambridge University Press.

Timmermans, S. and Berg, M. (2003) *The Gold Standard: The Challenge of Evidence-Based Medicine and Standardization in Health Care.* Philadelphia: Temple University Press.

Türkmen, S., Gillessen-Kaesbach, G., Meinecke, P., Albrecht, B., Neumann, L.M., Hesse, V., Palanduz, S., Balg, S., Majewski, F., Fuchs, S., Zschieschang, P., Greiwe M., Mennicke, K., Kreuz, F.R., Dehmel, H.J., Rodeck, B., Kunze, J., Tinschert, S., Mundlos, S. and Horn, D. (2003) Mutations in NSD1 Are Responsible for Sotos Syndrome, but Are Not a Frequent Finding in Other Overgrowth Phenotypes. *European Journal of Human Genetics*, 11: 858–65.

Turner, V. (1967) *The Forest of Symbols: Aspects of Ndembu Ritual.* Cornell: Cornell University Press.

Updike, J. (1998) *Bech at Bay: A Quasi-Novel.* Harmondsworth, Middlesex: Penguin.

U.S. Environment Agency (undated) What You Can Do to Protect Children from Environmental Risks. http://yosemite.epa.gov/ochp/ochpweb.nsf/content/homepage.htm (Accessed December 2011).

U.S. National Library of Medicine, National Institutes of Health. *Genetics Home Reference.* http://ghr.nlm.nih.gov/glossary=genotypephenotypecorrelation (Accessed October 2011).

Verran, H. (2011) Imagining Nature Politics in the Era of Australia's Emerging Market in Environmental Services Interventions, Special Issue: The Politics of Imagination, J. Latimer and B. Skeggs (Eds) *The Sociological Review*, 59: 411–31.

Wailoo, K. (1997) *Drawing Blood: Technology and Disease Identity in Twentieth-Century America.* Baltimore, MD: Johns Hopkins University Press.

Watson, M.S., Mann, M.Y., Lloyd-Puryear, M.A., Rinaldo, P. and Howell, R.R. (2006) Newborn Screening: Toward a Uniform Screening Panel and System – Executive Summary. *American College of Medical Genetics Newborn Screening Expert Group. Pediatrics*, 117, No. Supplement 3, May 1: S296–S307.

Webster, C. (1996) Medicine and Intellectual History: Intellectual History and Different Disciplines. *Intellectual News*, 1 (1): 34–5.

Wellcome Trust (2008) Research: 1000 Genomes Project. http://genome.wellcome.ac.uk/doc_WTX047611.html (Accessed November 2011).

Wellcome Trust (undated) Sanger Insitutute. Making a difference http://www.sanger.ac.uk/about/what/difference.html (Accessed March 2012).

White, P., Hillman, A. and Latimer, J. (2012) Ordering, Enrolling, and Dismissing: Moments of Access Across Hospital Spaces. *Space and Culture*, 15 (1): 68–87.

White, S. (2002) Accomplishing 'The Case' in Paediatrics and Child Health: Medicine and Morality in Inter-Professional Talk. *Sociology of Health and Illness*, 24 (4): 409–35.

Whiteford, L.M. and Gonzalez, L. (1995) Stigma: the Hidden Burden of Infertility. *Social Science and Medicine*, 40 (1): 27–36.

Willis, E. (2006) Introduction: Taking Stock of Medical Dominance. *Health Sociology Review*. Special Issue: Medical Dominance Revisited, 15: 421–31.

Wilson, P.M. (2001) A Policy Analysis of the Expert Patient in the United Kingdom: Self-Care as an Expression of Pastoral Power? *Health and Social Care in the Community*, 9 (3): 134–42.

Winter, R.M. (1996) What's in a Face? *Nature Genetics*, 12: 124–9.

Winter-Baraitser (2003) *Dysmorphology Database*. London: London Medical Databases.

Wynford-Thomas, D. (2003) How Long Should We Want to Live? Genes and Longevity. Panel presentation. *Genes and Society Festival*. Institute of Ideas. 26 April. Battersea Arts Centre, London.

Young, K. (1997*) Presence in the Flesh. The Body in Medicine*. Cambridge, MA: Harvard University Press.

Yoxen, E. (1982) Constructing Genetic Diseases. In P. Wright and A. Treacher (Eds) *The Problem of Medical Knowledge: Examining the Social Construction of Medicine*. Edinburgh: Edinburgh University Press. pp.144–61.

Zola, I.K. (1972) Medicine as an Institution of Social Control. *Sociological Review*, 20: 487–504.

Index

ROUTLEDGE INTERNATIONAL HANDBOOKS

Routledge International Handbooks is an outstanding, award-winning series that provides cutting-edge overviews of classic research, current research and future trends in Social Science, Humanities and STM.

Each *Handbook*:

- is introduced and contextualised by leading figures in the field
- features specially commissioned original essays
- draws upon an international team of expert contributors
- provides a comprehensive overview of a sub-discipline.

Routledge International Handbooks aim to address new developments in the sphere, while at the same time providing an authoritative guide to theory and method, the key sub-disciplines and the primary debates of today.

If you would like more information on our on-going *Handbooks* publishing programme, please contact us.

Tel: +44 (0)20 701 76566
Email: reference@routledge.com

www.routledge.com/reference

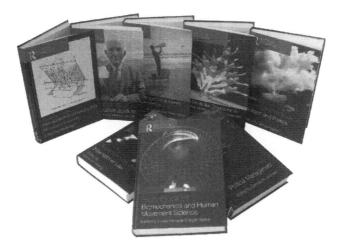

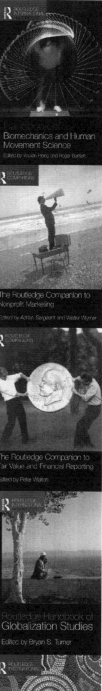

Biomechanics and Human Movement Science
Edited by Youlian Hong and Roger Bartlett

The Routledge Companion to Nonprofit Marketing
Edited by Adrian Sargeant and Walter Wymer

The Routledge Companion to Fair Value and Financial Reporting
Edited by Peter Walton

Routledge Handbook of Globalization Studies
Edited by Bryan S. Turner

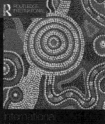

International Handbook of Sexuality, Health and Rights
Edited by Peter Aggleton and Richard Parker